Sacred Trust

The Ten Rules of
Life, Death, and Medicine

Phyllis Hollenbeck, M.D.

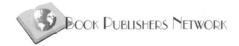
BOOK PUBLISHERS NETWORK

Book Publishers Network
P.O. Box 2256
Bothell • WA • 98041
PH•425-483-3040

Disclaimer—All names, except for those of my immediate family, have been changed.

10 9 8 7 6 5 4 3 2
Printed in the United States of America

LCCN 2005926803
ISBN   1-887542-25-6

Cover Design
Laura Zugzda

Editor
Vicki McCown

Interior Layout
Stephanie Martindale

To my sister, Meg—the One and Only

The Rules of Engagement

Preface

W hen my daughter was a baby in her stroller, wheeling around with me, people would stop us and say "Isn't she beautiful!"— and I would always say "And she's smart, too!" That baby girl with the gorgeous giggle also turned out to be very funny as soon as she got her hands on some words.

That's what medicine is: smart, beautiful and funny, all in one miraculous package. You can't take your eyes off it. And you shouldn't.

This book is for everyone to see what makes the world of medicine go round. Both for those officially in medicine, and those supposedly outside, these ten rules are a way to feel and think like a physician. It's a field guide to doctors—and it's a guidebook for life, with all its awe.

To me, these rules are also how healers happen, and why we all need it to happen right. None of my children are shrinking violets when it comes to voicing their opinions, and I'm sure they get some of that from their mother.

As one can say in anatomy class, see for yourself—it's all inside.

Acknowledgements

To acknowledge all who have stood with me in this work of the heart would be harder to do well than an Oscar speech. The names of these human beings are engraved both in heaven and on earth. They gave me platinum pieces from their lives, most precious and most holy—and for that I am forever grateful.

Rule #1
Being Human

I gimp along on the knee for six weeks. I am a fifty-three-year-old woman, a physician for twenty-seven years, and I do not like doctors. Most of them, anyway. The two nicest sentences that have been uttered to me in my career are "You don't look like a doctor" and "You don't act like a doctor." I always take those kinds of declarations as compliments at cocktail parties.

I like being a patient even less. The role of the patient means being infantilized, or worse, blown off by (usually) a guy wearing a white coat, whose training was essentially an enforced adolescence. He goes to medical school as a nerd and when he gets those magic initials after his name he becomes an eligible bachelor who still has no inter-human skills. Too many of these presumed geniuses should have done something else to make their parents proud.

"My God, my God, how soon wouldst thou have me go to the physician, and how far wouldst thou have me go with the physician?"

-John Donne,
Devotions, 1623

My left leg limp bothers my office mate, a good guy doctor, even more than it pains me. Tom is a man who writes plays and connects with his patients; as a pseudo-patient I present a definite challenge. After numerous days of watching me pull myself out of my desk chair and wince, he reaches the apogee of his annoyance.

"What the hell did you do?"

"Nothing. I sat cross-legged for forty-five minutes writing on my laptop and I had a little twinge when I unkinked my leg. It hasn't been the same since."

"What are you doing about it?"

"It's better with the knee strap and when I swallow the anti-inflammatory samples we have."

Tom makes a face like I do when I ask someone "How much do you smoke?" and they say, "Not much."

"You need to see an orthopedist. You've probably got a torn cartilage and it isn't going to sew itself back together."

This I know, and I also know that if weeks of what we call "conservative management" by a family physician (myself) hasn't gotten the swelling down or extinguished the searing pancake of pain right through the center of the knee that I enjoy every time I put direct weight on it, I need one of those surgical subspecialists to take a look.

"I'll just give it another couple of days," I say.

Tom looks as relentless as sin, even though his brother is the priest. "No—even if you can stand it much longer, I can't. You know you need an MRI and then an arthroscopy so somebody can go in and trim the damn thing."

I limp in and out of exam rooms four more times and come back to my desk to dictate. I feel the laser-guided spite of God boring down on me as soon as Tom walks back into our office.

"I don't want to see a jerk," I say.

"I know a good orthopod; he worked on my knee."

"You're still wearing a brace."

"I'm five years older than you are and so are my joints, and I could barely walk until he cleaned out my knee."

"How old is he? I don't want a boy doctor who looks like some student I've taught."

"He's got gray hair."

I rub my knee. "Does he know how to talk?" I ask.

"Yes. He's Irish. You'll like him—or you can come back and poison me."

The next afternoon, on my day off, I stand at the check-in opening in a wall on the other side of which sits a young woman. "I'm Dr. Hollenbeck," I say, "and I'm here to see Dr. O'Neill."

"Let me look it up." Her computer screen scrolls. "We have you seeing Dr. Harkins."

"No. My medical assistant made the appointment yesterday from our office and I know who I'm supposed to see. Dr. Palmero, whom I work with, specifically referred me to Dr. O'Neill." I smile.

"Well, I don't know who Dr. Palmero is. And Dr. O'Neill is all booked up. You'll have to see Dr. Harkins. He's really good with feet and ankles, and it's for your ankle."

"No. It's my knee."

"Well, you can reschedule."

"No, I can't. It hurts too much and I only have Fridays off and you have no idea how much it took to get me in here. And I know who I'm scheduled with."

We are at a healthcare standoff.

"Well, you'll have to see Dr. Harkins first and then I'm sure you can see Dr. O'Neill another time."

I smile. As my dentist says, smiling at people like this is what breaks crowns.

"I'm sure that after I see Dr. Harkins I'll want Dr. O'Neill to take a look at my knee before I leave."

She stares at me. The cursor blinks more naturally than she does. "You have to fill these papers out. And I need your insurance card."

"I don't have it yet; I just started with this group practice. But it's owned by the same people who run that big building you can see right next to us." I point out the window. "The hospital." She tries to look through me. "There are a lot of employees. I'm sure you've had other patients here with the same insurance."

"I don't know anything about these things."

At last—we are in total agreement. I limp to a seat in the waiting room, quickly fill out all the forms on the clipboard (thank

God I know the drill), and limp back up to the slot in the wall. Fifteen minutes go by and Ms. Receptionist finally calls my name and tells me I have to "go through that door to billing." More slow ambulation, but at least when I arrive on the other side the two young women there smile at me; maybe it's because they collect the money, but they also seem to know their job and look about ten years older than Ms. Receptionist.

"I don't have my insurance card yet."

"No problem. We can look up the group information because we see so many people who work there—and we have your social security number as the subscriber."

"My thoughts exactly. Thank you." I look at the billing slip: "Dr. Harkins." I tell them about the appointment mix-up and, no offense to Dr. Harkins, but I'm happy to wait to be worked in (and I'll add Dr. O'Neill onto my schedule if he ever has to be seen for acute bronchitis).

The brunette looks over the paperwork. "Oh. I'm really sorry to hear about the mix-up," she says. "Let me see what I can do."

Ten minutes later she spooks me while I am reading back in Ms. Receptionist's domain when she quietly crouches down next to my seat. "You're all set."

The woman who finally takes me back calls out only my first name as she guards the door to the royal chambers. She doesn't introduce herself until I ask her who she is. She says, "The doctor will be right in," which I know is a lie but I sit up on the table, dangling my legs and looking out at the roof of the hospital. I memorize the newspaper I have with me. Dr. O'Neill eventually comes in; he introduces himself and smiles.

"Thank you for working me in."

"No problem—I like taking care of people." Aha—a live one. He rolls his stool over to my knees. "This one is really quite swollen."

"It just looks that way from your level. Doesn't look so bad from the top down."

He pushes and pokes and I tell him it hurts right there. He gives me the verdict.

"You need an MRI, and if it confirms you have a torn meniscus you'll need arthroscopy sooner rather than later." He grins. "But only if you want your knee back."

I do. We talk about his wife who's a doctor but not working because she's taking care of the kids and she's fighting with her specialty board to extend her time frame to take the certifying exams until she returns to emergency medicine…and I tell him that a lot of women drop out because the system is set up for bachelors with slaves at home. He has to help me off the table and as I limp out of the exam room he says, "You can't wait another day to have this done."

Out in the hall Dr. O'Neill introduces me to Dr. Harkins who is immobile. He looks like he is sure I am a real estate agent and certainly never a doctor and his eventual handshake has less animation than those lifelike robots at DisneyWorld. My mother would watch his manners and ask, "Who brought you up?" I mentally thank Tom and the billing woman for saving me from the fate of being stuck with him.

In the course of my career in medicine I have decided it is not the gender of the doctor that counts but the degree of jerkdom. If it's tricky for me to find a physician whose brain crackles with the thrill of science and can also make a patient comfortable enough to be able to tell his story, imagine how hard it is for the average human being. Some people in the profession should not be there. Who lets these people in? Like clones like, so limited beings on medical school admissions committees pick their own kind because a candidate who uses both sides of her brain scares them and highlights their own shortcomings. And it is primarily men who decide who makes the cut—across the country, women do not often run medical schools, nor academic or clinical departments. I know this firsthand, having been "the first" or "the only" woman more times than I can stomach and from the stories of colleagues. Even men who combine art and science as physicians are often discriminated against; at a 250-physician group practice where I was the head of the family practice department, the guy whom I would have picked for my family was disparaged by the medical director as "not tough enough." This chief was someone who did not learn everything he was supposed to in kindergarten.

Medicine is a *service* profession. I believe this idea causes chest pain in many of my colleagues. Physicians are not so special that God likes to play "Doctor"; God or whoever or whatever decides who gets which DNA is the vehicle through which some human beings are blessed with the opportunity to take care of others. The practice of medicine is a sacred trust, and my heroes in it are Renaissance people—those intimately acquainted with the arts and scientific knowledge, who know that "history is 90 percent of the diagnosis," who understand that if you listen to the patient he will tell you what is wrong with him (this doesn't mean that someone will waltz into your office and say "I have a pheochromocytoma"), who taught me to take a history the way the famous Willie Sutton robbed banks—"because that's where the money is." They are clinicians who understand that if by the end of taking a history you have no idea what diagnostic bin the patient's complaints belong to, you're sunk—and that often when you open the exam room door you're facing a stranger, someone like all of us who does not want to be isolated in pain or fear.

It's "show time" when you cross that threshold and what you have to show is that you give a damn. Your first job is latching onto the telling phrase from the patient, because those words light the way to using your medical wits—not quickly scribbling a prescription or the acronym MRI. I remind medical students that they can only do a physical on a human in a few variations, as rarely does someone with dextrocardia arrive so they can listen to her heart sounds over the right side of the chest. But histories come in infinite forms. Over a hundred years ago the giants of this profession described many diseases (and yes, these illnesses are named after these dead white guys, but deservedly so) by using their brains to meticulously connect stories and then by the laying on of hands.

The definition of a good doctor is not "He's great at (1) cutting into you; (2) putting a tube up one of your orifices or into the arteries that feed your heart muscle; (3) treating your kidney failure." That is just "a pretty good doctor." The great ones are out there—I've been taught by them and taken care of by them. They read your face when you're in front of them and not just your EKG, and they consummately believe that this human behavior is not specialty specific.

Medicine still operates like a priesthood. Let me turn this on its ear—now that women are allowed to go to medical school the calling needs more "Sister Doctors," with the power to change the culture, as well as both male and female inductees who emulate them. This includes mimicking their usually much more legible handwriting. (Guess-what-I-mean orders, written in scribble resembling that of a drunken first-grader, can be dangerous to a patient's health.) Life has thrill and challenges and pain and undeserved suffering and that is what patients carry with them—they need complete caring as well as any possible cure.

In 1977 I wrote the essay for my yearbook at Brown Medical School and quoted Stephen Paget in *Confessio Medici:*

"Surely a diploma, obtained by hard examination and hard cash, and signed and sealed by an earthly examiner, cannot be a summons from heaven. BUT IT MAY BE."

No exclusive religion is required to believe in both the intangible as well as the technical and to be the conduit of that to a fellow human being. The education I sought out and found, my longing to learn, my need to always observe and understand—and serve—have given me guiding "Rules of Life, Death, and Medicine" that have stood me in good stead throughout my career. They are tenets that all those who aspire to this profession should know and never forget, that all students of medicine must live by. And anyone who has ever been a patient, or loved someone who has been one, or will be a patient, must understand these rules; for we are all "students of medicine" at some point in our lives.

I have been a witness and I ache to proclaim how to bring medicine back to its center. This is my story—and the rest of the rules.

Rule #2
They're Called Vital Signs for a Reason

Dr. Main stood by my desk and handed me a piece of paper. "I saw this lady today, and I ordered a CT scan and some lab tests ...you might hear about her on call tonight."

I smiled at him. Stephen Main was known for leaving each day before the stroke of five, so I considered saying "Nice of you to stay and risk turning into a pumpkin," but I behaved myself.

"What's her story?"

"She's forty-seven, new patient, I don't have any old records." He shifted his weight. "Five days of lower abdominal pain."

I scanned the faxed CT report: "...large transpelvic mass, ill-defined...abdominal and pelvic ultrasound to be done to further delineate its characteristics..." I clocked my eyes back at him. "What about her exam?"

"Not anything specific...but her abdomen was a little tight."

"Like an acute abdomen?" We both knew that meant a surgical emergency.

"No...just kind of hard." He swallowed. "I did a pelvic exam, but I couldn't find the cervix."

I let that hang in the air; I didn't ask him why he hadn't just come down the hall and asked me for help, especially since I did most of the women's care in our clinic. But I thought it.

Instead, I looked him over. "So what do you think?" I asked.

He didn't say a word.

I stayed at my desk a few more minutes to finish some dictation and then found Dr. Main's medical assistant and asked for Olivia Simpson's chart.

"How did this lady look, Tammy?"

She addressed the floor. "Not very good."

I examined the place in the chart where the vital signs are written. No pulse recorded, only one lonely blood pressure—of eighty over fifty.

"Did you do posturals?" I asked.

"No, I…I don't know what you mean."

I explained to her that checking blood pressure and pulse in lying, sitting, and standing positions could mean everything because of the information they carried. I told her not to feel bad about this and only silently wondered why Dr. Main hadn't taught her to use this tool.

The beeper went off with a call from Louise in the laboratory.

"Yes, doctor, I have a critical result."

"Let me guess—on Olivia Simpson."

"Bingo."

Olivia Simpson's white count was three times normal with a shift, which meant her immune system was sending in the type of white cells who act as the Marines and go in first to fight an infection; but her red blood cell count was only one third of what it should be. So I knew she'd been bleeding before today—or still.

"Is the patient there, Louise?"

"No, doctor…Dr. Main's order didn't say anything about that. But I have her phone number."

I got the voicemail voice. Fifteen minutes later Dr. Roberts paged me from radiology.

"I've got Olivia Simpson's ultrasound results," he said. "Hard to identify each part of the mass but her uterus is about twenty centimeters and it's full of pus or blood, or both." Now the white cells were mobilizing like a mob and swimming in a thick red sea inside a womb swollen like a pregnancy halfway to completion. But this was no baby; it showed only an ugly face.

"Do you know where the patient is?"

"No—but you could call out front to the check-in area. She was here with her husband."

They weren't there now. I alerted the triage nurse in the emergency room in case Mr. and Mrs. Simpson rolled in; I was afraid they were too polite and would sit quietly in the waiting room until her name was called. I tried the emergency contact number in the chart—busy four times.

Twenty minutes later the xray technician called me. Olivia Simpson and her husband had come back to the radiology department because they weren't sure what Dr. Main had wanted them to do.

"How do you feel, Mrs. Simpson?" I asked over the phone.

"Okay." She gave me permission to speak with her husband.

"How does she look to you?"

"Well, she was in a lot more pain several hours ago." *When she was in the office.* "But I think she's a little better now."

"She doesn't complain much, does she, sir."

"No. She hasn't been to the doctor since the birth of our child."

I told them what I knew and why I didn't want her to go home, and then I called the ER to let them know the patient and her husband were on their way downstairs.

Two hours later the telephone rang at home. It was Dr. Foster in the emergency room.

"I have Olivia Simpson here. I rechecked her red blood count and it's a little higher."

"That's because she's too sick to drink any fluids and getting dehydrated." Put the same amount of solid (red cells) in a shrinking volume of liquid (the blood plasma) and it'll look like it's a higher percentage of the container (the body). Falsely.

"She wants to go home."

"What's her blood pressure?"

"About eighty over fifty. But she's a small woman."

"Not that small; that's child size. She needs to be admitted."

"There aren't any beds."

We were only twenty miles from the next big city and not in Alaska. We didn't need a seaplane to get this woman to another hospital. I was beginning to think Dr. Foster was not in command of all of his medical faculties.

"Look. Pus—blood. Neither of them are good and we have no reason to think that either one of them have stopped. Call gynecology and have them put her on their service."

I hung up and went to bed secure in the belief that Olivia Simpson was where she belonged.

At twelve-thirty the next day our secretary Elizabeth stood at my office door.

"Dr. Hollenbeck, that lady you were so worried about from last night is on the phone; she says the pain is a lot worse."

"She's calling from her hospital bed?"

"No, she's at home. Her husband's with her."

I thought as I took a breath. "Tell them to get right in."

Olivia Simpson somehow walked in supported on the arm of her husband with their teenage daughter crying as she trailed them into the exam room. The patient's blood pressure lying down was eighty over fifty with a pulse of one hundred and ten beats per minute—the edge of the high normal range even though in that position her heart didn't need to strain against gravity to aim enough blood to her brain to stay conscious. When she sat up, her pressure slid to seventy over forty and her pulse jumped to one hundred and sixty-two beats a minute. I didn't try to stand her up again.

I nodded to my nurse whose hand had been on the phone to call 911 as soon as I had eyeballed the patient and had a few numbers to communicate. As two intravenous lines, oxygen and the EMTs went in, I asked her husband what had happened in the emergency room the night before.

"They told us to call for an appointment with the gynecologist this morning." He handed me a piece of paper—the discharge instructions from the ER. A computer-generated printout proclaiming a diagnosis of "abdominal pain," no closer to her precise, stealth danger than where he and his wife had started twenty-four hours before. "When I called this doctor's office today they told me she couldn't be seen until next week."

I reassured Mrs. Simpson's daughter that her mother wasn't going to die even though I knew that with the delay in care she was now one day closer to it. At the emergency room her mother spiked a temperature of 103 degrees Fahrenheit, was given three liters of intravenous fluids and four liters of "crystalloid" (a liquid specifically designed to keep her blood vessels open), and transfused with two units of blood. All this was necessary because she was in septic shock, a condition that had been cooking all this time, and a critical situation in which bacteria overrun the bloodstream setting off a cascade of chemicals that make (1) blood vessels leak so (2) blood pressure in the tubes plummets so (3) life-meaning blood flow to all vital organs shuts down, and at the same time (4) riotously consume clotting factors so that the patient concurrently bleeds to death. A trapeze act of exquisitely choreographed chaos that would be a diagram of wonder were it was not so life-stealing still—even—in modern hospitals.

This time a different ER doctor asked a different obstetrician-gynecologist to come in; after hearing her status, the specialist pronounced the patient "too ill to stay at our facility." *Now she was.* Mrs. Simpson was transferred directly to the intensive care unit of the nearby university hospital; the next morning, as soon as she was stable enough, the doctors there drained almost a liter of pus from her uterus, enough to nauseatingly fill a big bottle of soda. She "made it," surviving this perfect storm of destruction, only because she was just forty-seven and otherwise healthy until it hit her.

What went wrong? How did this "near-miss" happen? The picture was present from the beginning, but the doctor who saw this patient first didn't look or listen (nor did the second). Early in my career, a professor at Brown Medical School told us, "Your job is to know who's sick and who isn't"—and we thought he was a fool. But, of course, he wasn't; he was someone who knew how to nail a simple truth and hold it up for us to see, because someone's life would one day depend on it. Know the mechanisms of the body like beloved music, like learned prayers; know the paths and progress of diseases. Know these so well that you know what can wait and be attended to over time, and what is exploding before your eyes, eyes that see under the skin. Know what the patient may not be able to say—conscious or not.

Thus in my work I care closely for my patients, at that line where they count *as much* as my family even though they are not related to me by blood or law, ever vigilant for the one who could slip through my hands. The practice of medicine is that serious, and you never know when *that* person will walk in. Before every visit is over you have to stop for a moment and ask yourself, "Did I do my best with this human being? Did I listen for that bell in my conscience that says I heard why she came to me, and does she know I heard?" This isn't always easy, or possible, and it can't always be finished in one encounter—but it is the prize on which to keep your eyes. It means wanting to stretch your mind around what doctors call the "chief complaint," the patient's ticket of admission to your office, and stopping for that moment, to hear that sound in one's heart and mind, can make all the difference. For the bell that clangs back and forth between need and response is one that tolls for each of us in this existence, before the one, as John Donne wrote, that peals at the time of our death. It is the sound of hoping to stay connected to life.

So five women a day can come in with abdominal pain (and they do sometimes, because one of my minor rules is that things come in bunches, and there is always an unadvertised daily clinic special). How do you find "the one"? The first thing that each of them gets is all four vital signs: respiratory rate, temperature, blood pressure, and pulse, (and the recent, important addition of the assessment of pain on a scale of one to ten). Why are they called "vital signs"? Because they are the large objective measures of the life functions of the body—and thus their loss is also the way a doctor pronounces the moment of death. These numbers immediately tell a physician whether the body is under stress, and they are the first language and physical skill a medical student learns. Without expensive and invasive tests, with only the "technology" doctors had over one hundred and fifty years ago, taking these signs and knowing how to interpret them immediately tells you a great deal about the person in front of you. Analyzing them will direct your questions to gather more facts, even ones that the patient may not know are important. As was emphasized to me and as I have passed down to medical students, ignore these signs and their messages only at your patients' and your own peril.

On a basic level, vital signs can almost clinch a diagnosis because of their interrelation, but only if the clinician can read their elegance. They dance together. Fever raises pulse, but so does blood loss or dehydration, which eventually drops blood pressure; pain raises blood pressure and pulse and often how quickly someone breathes, but doesn't always come with fever. The reasons for the changes in vital signs must then quickly be sorted through, and the experienced clinician then notes which of them are running together—if it's fever and pain with normal blood pressure with or without changes in pulse, then you go in the direction of serious infection and sprint towards the lungs if the patient also has a cough; if there's no fever and the pulse is high with the blood pressure becoming low, with or without pain, or a change in respiration, think first of internal bleeding and/or that the patient has been too weak to take in enough fluid—and flush out the villain behind these scenes. On the other hand, a patient with no fever but a low pulse and blood pressure who is short of breath can be having a heart attack, with cardiac muscle that's dying and now can't pump well, even if he's in denial and doesn't want to acknowledge that big circus animal who is sitting on his chest. The interpretation of vital signs can even point toward one of the trickiest diagnoses in clinical medicine, referred to in a classic article as akin to the emperor who has no clothes, because it is often the one that no sees: pulmonary embolism (blood clot to the lungs) which can present without fever, with normal blood pressure but a rising pulse, and pain with breathing. And ever-present, often overarching all the "pure" bodily responses to attack, are the simultaneous reactions of the patient's mind, which can trump all.

Mrs. Simpson had a blood pressure of eighty over fifty, a number transparently lower than normal; she admitted to pain. A few simple questions would have elicited that she was stoic and probably downplaying her symptoms, but asking about her old records and finding out there weren't any would have confirmed just how much pain and fear it took to get her to come to a doctor. But even before all that, by checking her blood pressure and pulse in lying, sitting, and standing positions, just how ill she was would have been written in neon—because with gravity, if there is not enough fluid in the blood vessels, the heart will pump faster to get something to the brain, and this will be the first message before blood pressures in different positions start to drop. A large differential in pulse rate from one posture to another signifies a heart pushing for all its fame. It is the body shifting its gears so it will survive. Even if this lady was unwilling to admit to dizziness or being "sick," her numbers would have shouted it out.

Why didn't the first doctor to "see" the patient use all his wired organs to gather in all this information? It is the disconnection between knowledge and sense. In the exam room a week before another patient had voiced just such a breach to me.

"I saw Dr. Main once for bronchitis and that was okay. But a month later, at a routine check-up with my hematologist, my blood pressure, for the first time in my life, was 190 over 110. Even I knew that was sky high and they sent me right over from the office. Dr. Main came in and looked at my chart.

'It's a lot higher than the last time I was here, or any time at Dr. Walker's office,' I said.

'Right.'

'What do you think is going on?'

'I think you're just anxious, that's all.'

'Of course I'm anxious! You would be too if your blood pressure shot up like this for no reason!'

"I wanted to punch him. He sat there looking at me through his beady little brown eyes and I thought, 'You really don't care, do you?'"

Caring. That's it. It is the penultimate vital sign, without which the others are useless. You sit in the exam room with a doctor and your unspoken words are "*Help me.*" Tell me that everything is all right—whether I'm here for a yearly physical or a check-up for my heart, my diabetes—my cancer. If something is not right, tell me what we can do. Help me tell you that the masked worry over my strained marriage is what's "eating at me," and needs one treatment, while the crater it's burnt in the lining of my gut is visible and needs another. And when there is nothing more "medical" to do, tell me how to face that. And don't leave me. Don't leave me alone.

The cleavage starts when the doctor doesn't *care.* All of us as physicians are human and so any one of us, on any given day, can be tired or distracted or angry but below all that must course that abiding caring that pulls us back to why we are in that room with a patient. We must pick the right kind of person for this job; someone with the drive towards, the delight in, the feeling of satisfying service in getting to the heart of the matter with another human being. And, especially in a family physician, some-one who is not afraid to be Harry Truman and say, "Yes, the buck—the search—stops with me. Your search for an answer often will end with me because I will listen and use my hard-won skills and my *interest* to give you your diagnosis; and your search for a guide and an advocate and a partner in the healthcare maze will also end at my door."

This job requires a person of restless passion, diving into science as she swims towards a fellow human being in need. Someone who likes problems—preventing, understanding, and solving them—and is fearless in attacking them. Someone who gets a thrill and has an eternal fascination with figuring out people—both their human bodies and their human minds. I do not believe that drive can be taught; it can only be honed and polished. It must be there in the beginning in the person chosen for that seat in medical school. It must be someone who takes care in the present while looking into the future for what is planning ahead—what bacteria now multiplying, as he speaks to a patient, are behind that vague symptom of abdominal pain and tonight will strike like a torch in the blood; what lipid number on a page signifies that one day, five years from now, a shard of cholesterol will attach to an inflamed sore in the wall of a coronary artery and a clot will seal them, and this man in front of him will stop speaking to his wife in mid-sentence and drop dead. As none of us has a direct line to God, a physician cannot always make a difference; but wanting to know, deeply, the mechanisms of health and disease and of being human and not slapping that knowledge aside allows us to make all the difference we can.

This is not banking—where the to and fro of money can always fix a mistake (and the hours are better). This profession requires more than brains. When you hold a chart in your hands you hold a book of vital information that belongs to the patient, that together you add to, and that you explain and watch over; for when you open that door to the exam room you hold a person's life in your hands. All continuing and comprehensive care follows from that one moment of recognition. That seat in medical school is reserved for the one who can see this.

Three weeks after Mrs. Simpson's journey, Tammy stood at my desk at five-thirty.

She handed me a piece of paper.

"Dr. Main saw this man at two o'clock and he was in a lot of pain so Dr. Main ordered this blood test stat…but he's gone already…and this is really abnormal and I don't know what to do with it."

I wasn't on call this night but I knew I had to check the lab result. This time the white blood count was a little bit lower than

Mrs. Simpson's had been, but still whistling along that stairway to heaven.

"Let me see the chart."

"Dr. Main ordered a CT scan, too."

"For when?"

"Tomorrow."

I sat there for a minute and thought. I was on my way out the door. This was not my patient. Give it to the guy on call, or call the patient? Crap—call.

"Mr. Whelan, this is Dr. Hollenbeck. I work with Dr. Main and I have your blood test results from today." I scanned the scribble on the page—forty-three-year-old-male, fireman. Skinny chart. The last time he'd come in was three years prior to this and he'd waited it out for two weeks with a "cold" that was pneumonia. "Is the pain still in the lower right side of your abdomen?" I asked.

"Yes."

"For twenty-four hours? Pretty bad, huh?"

"Yeah."

"Do you still have your appendix in, sir?"

"Uh huh."

"I want you to go right into the emergency room. I don't want you to wait for that scan until the morning. I think your appendix will rupture by then."

"Okay."

Okay. No argument from a man—a MAN (the species that would rather die than come in; and, unfortunately, often get their wish)—someone who hardly ever went to the doctor. The pain was that bad; Tammy said he'd walked out of the office "pretty slowly." All he'd wanted was "permission" to go to the hospital because the doctor said it was serious. It was "bad" enough to order the blood count immediately but not "bad" enough to get the xray done right away. Was the patient "sick" or not? The differential diagnosis wasn't even as tricky as the possibilities with Mrs. Simpson: a man has one less organ system below the belt.

This is a cautionary tale. You see what you want to see. Dr. Main "sees" someone every ten minutes, up to forty people a day (I will address later why that number is rewarded). But you can quickly assess someone, as they do under more stress in emergency rooms, if you look first for what's vital.

Later that week a woman sitting in one of my exam rooms related the tale of her mother's recent trek through healthcare. She finished her story, looked at me, and said:

"To be a patient these days you have to pray."

Amen.

Rule #3
Speak the Real Language

"Your father hasn't urinated in three days."

"What?"

"I don't think he's been able to empty his bladder since Sunday. He seems like he's in a lot of pain, but you know him, he won't admit it."

"How do you know he isn't going?"

"He disappears into the bathroom and stays a long time and when I stand outside the door I don't hear anything. Then when he comes out he doesn't look very happy." She almost laughed. "You know that look."

"The plagued Boston Red Sox fan."

"Yes." We smiled at each other over the telephone line. "But last night all he did was keep getting up to try again and again. And—he left the toilet seat up."

I had my feet up on the desk in the doctors' lounge at the emergency room where I was working in upstate New York. I swung them down and impaled a pen into different days of the blotter calendar. I managed to hit a bull's-eye through the uninspired medical graffiti onto every shift I had until the end of the month.

"Cripes, Mum. He needs to go to the doctor. Today."

"He won't go."

"Let me talk to him."

My eighty-two-year-old father was six hours away in Massachusetts and hard of hearing, but I could have been standing six inches from his face and it wouldn't have made one atom of difference in how much he was listening to me now.

"I'm alright."

"No you're not."

"I just need to drink more water and it'll be fine."

"Drink more water and your bladder will burst."

"You're wrong."

"Which one of us went to med school?"

My mother got back on the phone. "He's standing here; actually he's standing here bent over, but he's shaking his head no and making a face at me." She paused. "And he's just pulled out his hearing aid."

Hah—he could try any tactic, but it would fail. For I am my father's daughter, and he knew it; and he was frightened and I knew that, too. He hadn't been in the hospital since World War I. The man who bought me ladder trucks, and dolls, and told me I could be anything I wanted didn't want to believe his body was letting him down in something he'd taken for granted since he was a child.

I called the visiting nurse association and Sharon went to the house on the order of my father's "local" physician (me). "She charmed him," my mother reported, and his next visit was to the emergency room. There the "nice young doctor" marshaled a catheter past a prostate clamped like a giant fist around the bladder neck and drained urine that was dammed up above his umbilicus. My father said he was ready to go home.

But he had to take a leg bag attached to an indwelling catheter with him or the channel would close and he'd be right back where he started—a leg bag that was mandatory, in command, and capricious. When he turned over in bed it often yanked itself free of the tube so it could baptize him with urine, a ritual that was both an indignity and a cavalier reminder that he wasn't the same man that he was before he became a "patient."

I couldn't get any time off so I monitored my father's care over the phone with the urologist, Dr. Jasper, trained in Virginia with an accent to match.

"He's got a huge prostate. I don't think I'll be able to get enough of it with the first procedure."

"I know." I knew. My mind clicked through the textbook: all those trips in the car when we had to stop frequently so Daddy could use a men's room; being in my bedroom in high school and hearing the frequent sound of our one toilet flushing during the night, followed by my father's *sotto voce* "Goddammit!" as he felt and stubbed his way back to the bedroom in the dark. (No illumination allowed because "I don't work for the electric company!") My father's prostate gland had been growing as my sister and I were—this medical event had been in rehearsal for probably twenty years.

"Besides, he's over eighty," the doctor from Virginia said. "His heart will probably give out before this gets him."

"He isn't planning on it."

Dr. Jasper's appraisal that "this" (the cancer) wouldn't "get" (kill) my father, was based on the statistic that 95 percent of men who make it to eighty have at least a microscopic focus of prostate cancer, reassuringly found on autopsies for deaths from other causes—with heart disease number one on that hit parade. But my father was on no heart or blood pressure or other drugs; he was smart enough to know his prostate was a problem, but he hoped he could outlast it. And he hadn't put a name on it.

I put skin back together with sutures, saved lives, and stamped out disease in a small way in a New York emergency room the day my father's surgery was scheduled. Dr. Jasper scraped out as much of the gland as was safe at one time from this unconscious man. My mother was at the hospital every day and as soon as my father was able, walking with him and his new leg bag to the solarium at the end of the hall. On the day of his discharge that is where Dr. Jasper found them.

"Mr. Hollenbeck, you can go home today." Dr. Jasper was standing at the threshold of the solarium, ten feet from his patient.

"What?"

"He has a hearing aid," my mother explained. She turned to my father and put her hand on his shoulder. "Leland, the doctor says you can go home today."

My father nodded at Dr. Jasper and smiled. "Am I okay?"

"Well, YOU KNOW YOU HAVE CANCER, DON'T YOU?"

That loud, from that far away, in front of three other patients and their families. To my mother the details of that scene were as permanent as a painting.

"Your father sat there stunned. And embarrassed. Jasper never moved an inch closer." Oh yes—the southern gentleman to the end.

My father came home and learned to live with his leg bag. I came home and whenever I brought up the idea that having another surgery would mean he wouldn't need the catheter anymore, he would slap his hand down on the kitchen table and say, "No more goddamn doctors!"

Instead, I went back to the hospital and looked at his bone scan with the radiologist.

"Are you sure you want to see this?" he said.

"Yes." The scientist needed to see.

"The cancer's everywhere, you know—all through his spine and hips. It was from the first time he came in."

I knew; Jasper knew. *"His heart will probably give out before this gets him."* Not in a man with "a heart like a hotel," as my mother put it, "room for everybody," and not in a man with clean coronaries by EKG, weight, and cholesterol numbers, and no medicines and no chest pain. Jasper still wanted to say he "knew better"—but only a presence like God can know what will go first.

In the last week of his life my father and I were sitting on the couch laughing at silent Laurel and Hardy movies. He got up to go to the bathroom and I rose as a sentinel, as he was a thin specter of himself. He came out of the bathroom and pointed to the leg bag that had followed him everywhere.

"There's blood in it."

I nodded.

"I have cancer, don't I?"

I nodded again, this time with tears in my eyes, and put my arms around all that was mortal and left of him.

Tell the truth—that is what a writer must do, and also the doctor. Each must choose words precisely, knowing what to say and when and how; and each must always think of the effect on the audience. Timing is everything; the audience must be ready for what you have to say. You don't ram it at them without preparation anymore than you do that pushing a cysto-scope into a bladder.

Each person who picks up a book, just as each person who comes to a doctor, is unique and brings his own satchel of hope and fear and memories and experience and education with him. This is the arena in which he hears the words. This is the place that the doctor steps into when she speaks. What bounces off one person can explode like a bomb in an undefended place in the heart of another—or make no sense at all to someone else. There is a way to tell someone anything, but it cannot be done in selfish haste anymore than a work of fine literature can be rushed to conclusion. The novice in each field must observe those who have the skill, want to echo this aching beauty, and then practice. Practice.

My father was intelligent and understood what was wrong with him, but to a man of his generation the word "cancer" meant death without rescue or reprieve. But even worse than the diag-nosis was the cruelty of how it was yelled across a room at him—the doctor not stopping to watch the face of the human being who was the target. Words hurled like swords, bullets with no backstop. Why go back to someone like that? Why listen to him ever again?

Why would a doctor ever do that?

When you know as a physician you will be the bearer of bad news, remember that the person to whom you bring it must also "bear it." Before you go to that person, stand still for a moment

and with the soul that is yours ask for the right words. Those
words will come. Bring those words slowly with you to the
human being whose mind is already racing ahead. Whatever you
must tell, sit with this human being, look in his eyes; do not flinch.
His pain is greater than your discomfort.

Those actors who play doctors on TV come out to the family in the waiting room, say, "I'm sorry," and then turn and disappear—I do not know how to do that and if you are in the right job
your legs will not walk you away. Perhaps you will need to be a
wailing wall; perhaps you will just be quiet with their tears; perhaps you will need to repeat the news in a different way. Again.
And again.

If you have done your best for the patient you will be able to
handle any question, the plan for what to do next, what something means, or doesn't. Some pleas will be unspoken, commu-
nicated only through the eyes, by an expression on a face. In
Raymond Carver's poem, "What The Doctor Said," a man
receives the news from his physician that his lung tumors are
back, and it is clearly painful for the doctor to say; yet the man
"hears" the wish to comfort and ends the poem remembering, "I
almost thanked him, habit being so strong." So you will be
humbled by someone's simple gratitude that you are still there.
In those moments you represent a grand tradition of healers—
not people who cure all, but human beings who are blessed to be
able to bring small balm to another. As you do this, remember in
a cache of neurons in your mind that when it is your turn to be the
"bearer," you will want the kind of doctor you are striving to be.

A physician gains strength for those moments from the far
more frequent ways she talks with patients. You explain the
counter-current system of the kidney in one way to an engineer;
you describe the changes in the blood tests that measure renal
function from another angle to the amazing eighty-eight-year-
old woman—"Even a Mercedes wears out." Humor comes with
being human and can be the kindest way of being direct and clear.

To the patient who has just developed diabetes and asks where it came from, the answer is "It didn't fall from the sky—it's that good old American hand to mouth disease"; and then you tell him how you will help him help himself. To the twenty-year-old whose cholesterol profile is already planning to separate her from her future, mention that fast food places should just build coronary care units right next store to avoid the middle man and the wait. On my way out the door the last thing I say to a patient who is thinking of quitting smoking is "Every time you light up I want you to think of me"—with a smile. I tell her if she doesn't quit the cigarettes WILL WIN, and I can always fill her spot on my schedule with someone else, but I'd rather it was she because we've gotten used to putting up with each other. Or you might mention, in my mother's words, that if she keeps smoking she probably "won't make old bones." When the soccer player wants to know why the bruise he got on his knee is now "spreading" down his leg even as it mutates from purple to yellow, I explain "Gravity wins. Everything slides downhill," even ruptured hemoglobin in soft tissue. (I do not use physics in referring to any changes in women's anatomy over time, because I would strangle anyone who said that to me. Besides, bellies move on men). For the husband whose wife is with him to make sure she knows what I tell him ("Because he'll come home and say 'The doctor said everything is all right.'"), and he isn't taking his blood pressure medicine, just ask him if his life insurance is paid up and does he want his wife to be one of those merry widows dancing on a cruise ship. And using the quiet data on the laboratory report that shows how alcohol changes the way bone marrow produces red cells even before alterations in the liver functions, I ask the nervous young woman, "How much do you drink?" Once she gets past her surprise at my detective work, she answers, "Whatever it takes"—and I smile, thank her for her honesty and *her* humor, and the real dialogue begins.

But for "smack you on the head with a balloon reality", and keeping even your unvoiced communication clear, children win. I pride myself on explaining each part of a physical exam as I'm going along…"Swallow now, this is to check your thyroid gland"… and I always listen over the four cardinal heart sound areas as I was taught. (However, as swamped interns we wanted to inhale the temptation to use "Quickie's Point"—that spot just below the bottom of your breastbone where you can listen to the heart, lung and bowel sounds all at once, saving time—for sleep.) I thought I was being impressive and didn't think to explain this maneuver until the day I did a sports physical on an eight-year-old and was moving the stethoscope over his chest. He sat quietly, then looked up at me with a question in his eyes: "What's the matter, Doc, can't you find the heart?" His concern over just what kind of clown he was at the mercy of was pasted all over his face, as was the message, "Do you have any idea how this looks to a patient? Stop congratulating yourself, Doc, on being so complete if you haven't told me what I need to know."

Out of the mouth of a young partner—and don't you forget it. I haven't, ever since.

Knowing the real language and speaking it, understanding it, doesn't always mean in your native tongue. The first time I saw a patient in pain I was in a foreign country. In the summer between my junior and senior years at Brown University, I cradled my passport and flew overnight from Boston to Amsterdam. I traveled over water into the rest of my life, and every time I looked out the window of the plane into the cold blue of heaven I saw the world opening up to me. Instead of sleeping, I imagined lassoing a rope around *La Tour Eiffel* and pulling the plane faster to the continent.

The Dutch capitol was jammed with sun, honking toy cars, and background babel as people on bicycles threaded their way to Monday morning work, and I followed suit, pedaling immediately to my assignment at "Sint Lukas Ziekenhuis": Saint Luke's "Sickhouse." The hospital. I silently repeated this new poetry, aching for fluency in the universal, holy, world of medicine—for the rhythm of belonging.

I was sent to the kidney dialysis unit where a blonde nurse only a little older than my twenty-one years welcomed me with the musical precision of continental English. Leave your civilian habit behind and change like a willing nun, a soldier, into the required uniform of white scrub dress, white clogs, and kerchief head cover. The clear double doors of the unit slid apart into a gallery of stainless steel functions and white forms, sleek as a European kitchen on the other side of a looking glass. Manna. Professional efficiency breathed in and out in the space, all quiet background except for the soft mewing of a patient, skin stretched to translucent parchment, who was being helped onto the scales. Poor woman, I thought. How different from me.

Kidneys that failed her could not remember how much salt and water to hold onto, nor how much waste to filter from the blood, meaning that by the day of each dialysis she was bloated with a poison of her own making. I saw thin threads of hair hanging without order around her swollen face. I heard the sheets, fiercely pressed, scratch her body as the nurse pulled her onto the bed, and then the machine next to her began to whirr: *I'm here to save your life…aren't you lucky I'm here to save your life…I'm here to save…* The woman said nothing.

A man in a white coat arrived. He snapped on sterile gloves as the nurse unwrapped a green package on the tray next to the bed, revealing two large needles with slanted ends. They commanded center stage among the instruments, reflecting the overhead light; they shone like polished spears.

"What are they for?" I whispered to the nurse.

"One is for the artery, and one is for the vein; that's the way the doctor will hook her up to the machine. They go into the fistula under her skin."

"Where's the fistula?"

"Right there…on the inside of her wrist." She pointed to a thick snake, bulging as it strained against its cover.

I nodded as I puzzled this out. The fistula was a surgical site where an artery and vein had been connected. That double conduit made it possible for the dialysis machine to take the patient's blood from her artery, run it through the cleaning cycle, and return it through the tube connected to her vein.

The inside of the woman's wrist was swabbed with iodine, and the nurse held her elbow and hand. Down. The woman looked at me. The doctor handcuffed her with his left fingers as his right grip bore forward with the large needle under the skin. The woman twisted, the weapon slipped—and as the patient screamed a fire hose line of red shot out onto the field of white. I forgot the time zones I had crossed and that I hadn't eaten any breakfast as I stood watching, transfixed. With the overhead light swinging and the floor rolling under my feet.

I fainted.

I awoke to a circle of faces chattering in Dutch, then smiling at me. I swished the blood off an edge of tooth, drank some orange juice for blood sugar, and then went to the bed of the woman. She was "attached" now and her eyes were closed. She opened them, caught mine, and then went back behind her eyelids again. I couldn't hear her breathing over the noise of the machine, but I could see her name and her age on the clipboard at her feet. Kaatje was just eighteen.

Illness had stolen time from her as it aged her beyond her years. Now I knew what she had been saying as she tried to wrestle out one more moment of freedom before being chained again to a box outside her body: *Why me?*

I only had to look to speak her language.

Rule #4
I Told You
What I Told You

"Okay. Tell me again where the pain is; point to it with one finger."

Mary O'Shea and I were facing each other, she perched on the side of the stretcher and swinging her legs in front of me on my stool. "A cooperative adult female looking at least her stated age," in the classic opening syntax of a medical case presentation. This female was outfitted in the oversized bib of a hospital gown with only a curtain screening off her naked spine from the audience of other victims in the emergency room. Mary fidgeted with the momentum of a child aching to give me the right answer even though a few minutes ago, as I had leaned over her to lay my hands on her abdomen hoping to divine the source of her pain, the leftover perfume of tobacco had climbed into my nose.

I was working a Friday night shift in the local hospital where I was on staff. Mary and I knew each other from the occasions when I was up in labor and delivery as a young family physician managing to follow the lead of a slippery newborn in one of the rooms that she cleaned. She always wore a loose green scrub dress under an operating room gown when she swished her way around her usual neighborhood, making everything she touched disappear—blood, mucus, amniotic fluid and/or the occasional soupy remnants that had made a reverse trip up from the stomach. No matter what she discovered, Mary smiled as she went about her chores. She and the nurses and I constituted the female working brigade in that department, and right now, from the neck up, Mary looked the same as yesterday.

I had told her it was fine to keep her socks on and now she crossed those red wool ankles and looked down at her overweight stomach, finally pointing to a spot halfway between her belly button and her pubic hair. "Right here," she said.

"What did you eat for dinner?"

"Meat and potatoes—like always. And I had one beer. That's all."

I looked at my notes on the ER sheet. "So how long after that did the pain start?"

"Oh, the pains started before that, when I was still at work, but then they started to come more regular."

"How regular?" We'd been down this line of questioning before, and now I felt like I was circling a drain. It was close to midnight. But I smiled as I shoved my fingers into my left temple. "Give me a ballpark of how regular—everybody's got a different definition of that."

"Oh, you know—like cramps." Mary smiled back at me.

"From gas?"

"No. Like a period."

"When was your last period?"

"It just ended."

"And you haven't missed any?"

"Nope."

"And it doesn't hurt to urinate?" She shook her head. "No fever or chills?" Another shake. "So are you nauseous?"

"I was a little bit in the beginning."

The beginning…in the beginning…the beginning of what? I ran through the major organ systems in the lower female trunk: guts, bladder and kidneys, and gynecological. The history didn't fit with a stomach flu, or appendicitis, or a urinary tract infection or clot to the bowel circulation, or a hernia, and on a dare she hadn't swallowed a pen refill that was now stuck midway to the exit ramp (that had been the fourteen-year-old male on my last night shift)…and she was forty-three, not sexually active, with no family history of ovarian cancer and no irregular vaginal bleeding, but she hadn't had a Pap smear in years and she did feel a little bloated…I was going to have to do a pelvic exam.

I stood up and stretched. I told Mary the plan which meant moving her to a room with a door for some measure of privacy. But before we did that I decided to go back to basic medical student training and give getting a working diagnosis one more shot.

"Mary—if you had to describe the pains in your own words, what do they feel like?"

"Well, I've never been pregnant," she said, "but I think this must be what it feels like for those women I see in labor." Swell, I thought, she's a big help.

The nurse stood at the head of the exam table holding Mary's hand as one of the cramps came, and I rolled my stool up to her draped bottom. I lifted the sheet as I told Mary what to expect next, and then I stopped talking. I peeked over the drape and crooked my finger at the nurse, motioning her to come look—for there, in between Mary's thighs and ready to burst in my face, was a bulging bag of water and a baby's head right behind it. And now the whole balloon was sliding towards me as Mary made a little moan.

The nurse called to alert labor and delivery that we were on our way and I got Mary's feet out of the stirrups, put her knees together, and took her hand. "You're about to have a baby," I said.

"I am?"

"No doubt about it." I smiled. And Mary smiled back the way I imagine another "virgin" finally did at the announcing angel.

But my Mary had become a mother doing something "good Catholic girls don't do"—so she proclaimed her news to me in her own code.

Several years later, on a routine afternoon, a thirty-two-year-old woman came to my solo private practice. Thank God I now had a little more "practice" in my bones and in my brain. I read her answers to the new patient intake questionnaire, noting that her chief complaint was "abdominal pain that came and went," and we began.

"You're the fourth doctor I've seen for this."

Uh-oh. Bad sign—three up, three down. Each of those other members of my profession had passed the audition, done an acceptable song and soft shoe in rehearsals, and then flopped on opening night. Was the director looking for only-in-the-movies perfection (aka "doctor shopping"), or had none of the others understood how to play their part?

Or—did the script only exist in the director's head?

I smiled back at Ms. Cavanaugh. She looked normal. Classy professional jacket and skirt, simple pumps, handbag more well-behaved than mine. Make-up applied like a magazine shoot; lipstick certainly not swerving off the mouth rails in what we'd been taught was the way of the hysteric.

"Hysteric," of course, meant belonging to, or suffering in, the uterus—an organ that only women had. Hysteria was taught to generations of medical students as a disease "peculiar to women," one with physical symptoms that could not be attributed to any bodily pathology. No one was able to find the cause of this patient's pain; I hoped her uterus wasn't blocking anyone's view of the dialogue.

In those first few moments of thinking, luckily, I remembered the psychiatry professor at Brown who said: "Crazy people don't die of being crazy, they die from the same things you and I do." And the other teacher who said: "No matter what some prior physician has said, or the diagnostic label the patient drags into the room with them, make sure it makes sense to you. When that patient is in front of you—think for yourself."

I decided that as much as we all want to be "the hero doctor," I might not make a diagnosis that someone else missed—but I had nothing to lose by trying, and this woman would at least have a chance for something gained. This was a real patient. I could be the real doctor Brown trained me to become, and that I hoped I was.

"I hope you can help me." Ms. Cavanaugh leaned forward towards me, and the exam table paper buckled. "I can't take this much longer. I know something's wrong."

I aimed my pen to take notes. "Well...just start at the beginning and tell me the story. I'll look at the old records you've brought after that."

The pains seemed to come on suddenly, but sometimes didn't come until eight hours after a meal; they could wake her from a sound sleep, and last minutes to an hour, waxing and waning in severity. The last time she'd had them was four days ago. She didn't run a fever with them, or develop a rash, or puke, or have the rapid transit diarrhea that my mother called "the green apple quick step;" and no other specific food seemed to trigger them. They weren't related to her period, or get any worse when she was pregnant. The only thing that made them go away was time, and trying not to move. She still showed up for work every day. No one else in her family had ever had anything like them, no one knew what to call them—and whatever they were, she'd had them occasionally ever since childhood, but they hadn't killed her yet. And she hadn't lost any weight, or developed any other symptoms that ran in tandem with them. How bad could whatever this was be? Fluttering at the edge of my medicine mind were the acronyms we'd used as residents lurching for a reason for symptoms such as these: "GOK" or BTHOOM"—God Only Knows or Beats The Hell Out Of Me.

The thing was, I also knew that a failure to find a diagnosis on our part didn't mean the patient didn't have one. Another medical acronym was "WNL," meaning "within normal limits" or nothing remarkable. We kidded that it could also mean "we never looked"—but right now, at least with Ms. Cavanaugh, that wasn't a very funny joke.

Nobody had looked.

People listened to her, and then her bowel sounds, pushed on her abdomen and checked her pelvis. The histories taken and the blood tests done varied to a greater or lesser extent, but the one constant was exactly what she'd said to me: "The pain feels like something in the middle of my stomach twists, and then eventually untwists." I knew there was a condition known in children, called volvulus, which was just like this. Loops of small bowel could telescope and/or turn on themselves, because they were not as firmly "tacked down" to intra-abdominal connective tissue. The pain was excruciating, of sudden onset and variable duration, but resolved on its own as long as the self-applied anatomical "tourniquet" unkinked before the blood supply to the unlucky intestinal site was cut off long enough for tissue to start dying.

This problem wasn't supposed to happen in adults (see rule to come). But it fit her description, in her own words, perfectly; and if that is what was happening, and just one time she got unlucky enough to have that "twist" stay stuck, she'd be on her way to the operating room to have rotting guts removed—if she got lucky enough to have someone make the diagnosis of impending peritonitis in time. Once her insides burst and spilled what was inside them into her abdominal cavity, it would be a fight to the finish.

And the one fairly simple, and not too dearly expensive, (even in often highly priced medicine) test that would have at least given her the benefit of the doubt, and looked at the area in question, had not been ordered. Nor had any other of the then-available imaging tests been done. I rechecked her old records and asked her another question.

"Did you ever have any xrays, like an upper GI?"

"No. And I know what that is. I asked for it, and they said I didn't need it because it wouldn't help."

Fair enough—as far as that thinking went. It was unlikely that she had a "fixed," or stationary, narrowing in her digestive tract. The symptoms would come more often, and be related to putting something into the channel, as with eating. And things should occasionally come up or go out quickly, especially if whatever was causing the narrowing progressed, due to a traffic jam happening as the body tried to propel meal remnants forward and the loops of gut went into spasm as they squeezed. And she wasn't describing spasms—the pains didn't come in waves or migrate even a little. Another defect, possibly congenital, with a bulged out section of the intestinal wall acting like a pocket where partially digested food could get caught didn't completely fit the history either; because, like an appendix, that little alcove should eventually get inflamed enough to stay sore, accompanied by a fever or blood or other change in bowel habits. The "Upper GastroIntestinal" wouldn't clinch a volvulus diagnosis unless it "caught" the event happening at the same time the radoilogy movie was being filmed. But by trying to imagine a physical reason for what the patient complained of, and keeping an open mind, and believing her, "running her gut" filled with "contrast material" like barium would at least give us an outline of the highway—and it would rule out the other causes.

I started to fill out a radiology requisition. I put her symptoms down in "Reason for Procedure," and wrote "? Cause" under "Diagnosis."

"Okay," I said, "let's do an upper GI, with a small bowel follow-through. I'm adding that other test, because then the doctor in the xray department will have more pictures as the barium river leaves your stomach and travels down to the three parts of your small bowel. We'll see it in motion. That way we'll at least try to check-out one part of the body where your pains are."

Ms. Cavanaugh's shoulders fully relaxed for the first time since I'd opened the exam room door. "Thank you," she said. "Thank you."

I knew I'd also made it past the audition, and at least at this point, I was at the head of the chorus line. Except—where I went to school, the moves I was doing were considered the basic skills expected of all performers. The script I was following was only proper.

Ms. Cavanaugh's upper GI and SBFT were scheduled for two days later. Just after the appointed hour on the appointed day, my secretary Anne knocked when I was with a patient and said another doctor was on the phone.

"Who is it?"

"The head of the radiology department."

I picked up the phone. "Phyllis—Jim Vogel here. Phyllis—I have your patient Ms. Cavanaugh here, and you're not going to believe this…(I was)…but when we watched that barium enter and start to pass through her small intestine, all of a sudden one section seemed to telescope and twist up around itself and she said she got the same exact pain…"

Luckily, the density of the barium stream "pushed" past the volvulus area and moving like the front end of a smooth locomotive, dilated it and it untwirled like a telephone cord pining to resume its customary shape. Ms. Cavanaugh saw a surgeon who tacked all the parts down "for life," then came back to me in follow-up.

"You're a genius."

"No, I'm really not." But I could feel the bones in my skull moving ever so slightly apart as my head began to swell. I needed to sit on it.

"But you listened. And you believed me. It wasn't all in my head."

I smiled. "No—you felt it in your gut, both kinds. You knew it. And you were right. I just did my job."

There, that let a little air out of the inflated balloon on top of my shoulders, much as I hated to see it go. Besides, balancing a big head on a high pedestal is akin to an Olympic event and requires lifelong vigilance to maintain your position. You have to think only of yourself.

And even God doesn't do that.

My mother was a woman of brains, music, resolve and charm. She believed in the famous Virgin Mary (whom she quietly saw as the power behind the throne), and she believed in saying what she meant. In person she was five-feet-two, 115 pounds (except with two pregnancies), but you would have testified in court that 75 percent of that weight was due to her spine of steel. She was also the personification of Irish Diplomacy: "How to tell a man to go to hell so that he looks forward to the trip." If you came back to her trying to finagle a different answer over something you wanted to do (like take the car overnight) or didn't want to do (such as the dusting), she would smile and say, "I told you what I told you." End of story. Ask again, and she'd say the same words in the same sweet way again. When appropriate, she was immovable.

I've often thought of this trait of hers in my years as a physician, whenever someone tells me a story of serial doctors such as Ms. Cavanaugh's. I wish my mother could have been in the room with the first doctor and immediately injected the patient with a bolus of flint: *I told you what I told you. I meant it. Believe me.* Yes, there are patients who keep changing doctors, but we also know that most of them do it for one main reason: They don't feel validated. What they *feel* isn't being understood. Whether it's from the chest or arm, with anger or sorrow, their *pain* is real to them, and they need someone to acknowledge that. It's the same reason people fight over, and over, about the same problem in a family—you haven't got a prayer of it ending until everybody knows and believes that his or her point of view is being heard and considered in the final decision. Words are the only currency patients have. With all the patients you will see in a career in medicine, counterfeiters are very few.

But these two patients also reveal the other meaning of *I told you what I told you*: *I'm telling you what I have. I'm trying to help you; please help me.* Mary O'Shea could barely bring herself to look at her pregnant belly because she was over forty, and Catholic, and single, and drank and smoked and took high blood pressure pills and all these things were bad for babies so she couldn't be having one—but her lovely truth still came out just when it was needed. She told me the exact cause of her pains. My brain just needed to be open to "Why doesn't any of her history jive with any diagnosis?" (at least any of the ones I am thinking of), and my hearing only had to be alert to what she was actually saying. I should have stopped in my doctor tracks at the words "like those women in labor" and asked myself, "Why in hell would she put it that way?" Ms. Cavanaugh wasn't as shy or conflicted as Mary, but she had to keep repeating herself, because no one took her words seriously. Each of these women had a compelling voice. And both of these women enlarged my education, for like teachers of music, they helped train my ear.

I'm describing it the best I can—what could it be? Help me here.

Because it always *is* something; or as my mother would say, "If it isn't one thing, it's the same thing." (See family reference above). It's the same thing until you get to the bottom of it. The feeling of fatigue may turn out to be a silent attack on the fibers of heart muscle and/or the pain of a depressed soul, but enough engaged dialogue and the tests those words dictate will reveal that. The source will be unburied. The patient who calls every week with a new complaint as soon as you fix one problem is actually calling for the same reason—the need to be heard. "They enjoy poor health"—more of my mother's words—but they "enjoy" it only because it gives them the attention that is still missing in their life. They feel invisible. Figure that out, tell them they can have a regular appointment so you can "keep an eye on" them and their symptoms, and they will stop panicking about not being "seen."

Ms. Cavanaugh kept having to say the *same* thing—and she was right on the money. Her money, her body, her life. I wonder what she would have done if I had listened to her story and told her I couldn't think of anything to do. I hope she would have pole vaulted off the exam table, barred the door, and yelled "Think about what I told you I feel, and do something, because I'm not letting you out until you *do think*!" Because if I'd done the former, and she hadn't done the latter, I would have flubbed my chance to be a real doctor: One who takes another's currency, and makes it count.

I didn't want to tell either Mary O'Shea or Ms. Cavanaugh how close I could have come to not helping them. How being taught to not cut corners, even in a nutso emergency room shift, meant I checked all regions in Mary below the waist and didn't just tell her I thought it was probably gas. Listen—since you don't have it now, come back if it gets worse, or if you see something new. Which she would have. Shortly. And not everyone would have blamed me for missing a diagnosis—hell, you should have seen the surprised looks on the faces of all those OB-GYNs, doctors who had seen Mary every day up to delivery, when she showed off her beautiful baby girl.

And Ms. Cavanaugh—what if I hadn't thought for myself? What if I hadn't acted as if I were the first and only doctor she'd seen for her symptoms? What if I hadn't done the things that are truly "just part of my job"? But who would have blamed me—no one else "found" anything.

Faced with a patient, with a jammed office schedule, or an overflowing ER waiting room, what "saves" a physician? Symptoms, ideas, tests flip in your mind like results at the racetrack. On the tightrope of your daily work, how do you dare to stay upright and vow to make it across, time after time? How do you help the patient walk with you in what could be a life or death moment? The safety net will always be the right kind of schooling in the right kind of person—a person with a medical conscience, who will feel inescapably lousy if she doesn't give it her best, and teachers who are the same. Humans with an unwavering sense of where they stand. Professors who know and *love* the rules, who ache to pass them on with ardor and respect, who don't think they know it all but keep things in balance. Doctors who step back from a power struggle and look to themselves first to understand why they're in such a tug-of-war with the patient. Teachers who came to mind as different when I asked myself why no one had ever just ordered an upper GI on Ms. Cavanaugh. Was it because she asked for it? Did they feel shaky that she might level the playing field? They didn't have to try to save face. It wasn't going to be any skin off their nose—they didn't even have to swallow that chalky white stuff called barium.

Such things as those described above saved me, and I think of them as blessings (along with *both* my parents and the way they treated people). Take medicine seriously, take patients seriously, even though you can still both laugh out loud in the exam room. (There is no law against that). But remember you can never spend too much time going over a patient's history if you haven't gotten to the bottom of the problem, even if it means you do it in more than one visit, or the next morning when you're drinking coffee at your desk. Gnaw at it because it should gnaw at you, become stuck in your craw until you can yank it out. If after doing all the right steps you still can't put your arms around a diagnosis and dance with it, remember you can still say you believe what that patient is telling you and together you'll take this one step at a time. You will never go wrong wanting to believe what a patient is feeling or aiming to understand what he is trying to say. Even a patient addicted to opiates is trying to tell you something in the way he concocts his story asking for another prescription. And you are both served best when you pay attention to that.

They say the last doctor to see the patient makes the correct diagnosis, as happened with me and Ms. Cavanaugh, because the patient stops searching after that. Unfortunately, that also applies to pathologists, they who make a living by doing autopsies on the dead; they are said to know everything, but too late.

But no matter how you slice it, or who does it, this rule still applies:

Patients tell you what they tell you—and always for a reason. Your job is to find that keynote.

Make sure as a doctor you fully understand the job you've chosen to accept. Neither you nor the patient should be on a mission that's impossible.

Rule #5

Bodies Don't Read Medical Textbooks

I stood outside on the fire escape and looked out over the city. The hospital was high on a hill, and I was six stories up. Cool air, night horizon; 2 am. My stethoscope was slung around the back of my neck like a tired pet snake. I was twenty-six years old, wearing a rumpled blue scrub dress under a "white" coat which now charitably resembled "dove grey," its pockets jammed with tongue depressors, index cards for each patient I was responsible for (including the four new ones that I had admitted that night on call), a black box that had my number and went by the name of "beeper," and one of my accessory brains—*The Washington Manual of Medicine.* A how-to for the new-to-it. When someone's heart stopped beating and I ran to a Code Blue I had to hang onto everything for dear life. Literally. I had managed to wash my face, and swipe at my teeth with a brush, but like a marooned *Jeopardy* contestant, my answer to the question of sleep was, "What's that?" I already knew why they called what I was doing being a "house officer"; I lived here.

Beast of burden that I was, still I stood on that metal balcony with a smile on my face. I was where I wanted to be. A month ago I was a medical student—now they called me "Doctor." I was working on addressing myself that way.

I went back into the hospital to the fourth floor residents' lounge. Charlie Parrish, the third-year senior family medicine resident, was stretched out on the couch, watching a guy selling a gadget on television. He launched his signature grin at me as I sat down.

"I think I'll order that thing to take out gallbladders with," he said. "And don't you look glamorous tonight. How many so far?"

"Two heart attacks, one appendix, and a guy who fell off his ladder while painting his cathedral ceiling living room and fracture dislocated both elbows." I started to laugh—the way you do in church. I knew I was getting punchy.

Ever ready for one but not yet in on the joke, Charlie lifted an eyebrow. "What?"

"He picked a nice color."

"How do you know?"

"He walked in wearing most of it on his head."

Charlie swung his legs down, stretched, and stood up. "Well, sister, I'm going into the arms of Morpheus."

"Yeah. I think I'll get some sleep, too."

"Hey—not so fast, my pretty. The emergency room is going to call you whenever somebody rolls in who needs to stay at this inn, and that ambulance siren's song is going to repeat until dawn. So let's go over the three things you need to remember as a medicine plebe. First—everything you know is wrong; second—it'll get worse before it gets better; and third—who ever said it'll get better?" He walked over and put his hand on my shoulder. "And one more thing for tonight"—a wink—"don't kill anybody."

Okay. Rub it in. As we put in my medical school yearbook at Brown: "These here as is below ain't reg'lar thoroughbred Sawbones; they're only in training." Thank you, Charles Dickens and Charlie Parrish for capsulizing why patients are warned not to get sick in July when the new recruits start.

Charlie was one of the finest doctors I've ever known, and as my mother would say, he "had an answer for everything." When he got paged in the middle of the night to examine an eighty-year-old woman with Alzheimer's disease who had "Houdinied" herself out of her bed restraints and fallen, he told the night nurse his assessment: "A little old lady fell out of bed; a little old lady fell on her head. If she'd fallen any farther she would have been dead."

That meant his orders were: "Equip patient with parachute and crash helmet." When he managed to fracture a finger in the hospital softball game, the middle one, of course, he followed the instructions "keep it elevated" to the letter whenever he walked by the office of the director of the residency. He drove the Mother Superior who ran the hospital to wear out her knees—praying. But those of us in training idolized him.

And he taught us to think our way to the answer; or answers. Precisely. When you're a medical student and then a resident, you spend a lot of time pinballing between two thoughts (this is only after you've passed through the stage where you are convinced that each disease you have just studied is now tunneling its way through your own body): I'll never learn and remember all this stuff—and because of that someone will die. Charlie kept pulling the lever on us, keeping the little metal balls in our heads from sitting still, because he wanted us to become aces at the game. He trained us to be champions who thought of every possible move. The cartoon on his outpatient clinic office door was a tombstone with the name and dates of the deceased, and these words engraved underneath: *I told you I was sick.* You were allowed to sleep in snatches on a thirty-six-hour shift; but God help you if you rested because you were too lazy to think about why someone was sick.

It's a Tuesday night, six o'clock. Mrs. Shaughnessy is sitting propped up on the gurney in the emergency room, stuck to the bleating heart monitor, IV line in and oxygen flowing into her lungs through two attractive, one-size-doesn't-fit-all plastic prongs in her nose. Her husband Paul is sitting next to her, but both he and his chair are tap dancing less now that her pain has subsided. I am supposed to run this kind of case by the senior resident before discharging the patient. I call Charlie.

"What ya got?"

"A fifty-eight-year-old female who three hours prior to admission had the insidious onset of an aching pain in her right upper back, accompanied by shortness of breath and feeling light-headed. Maybe some sweats, she's not sure. She was just sitting down to dinner, hadn't done any extra work that day, never had this before, pain never radiated, but waxed and waned until her husband drove her here…no past medical history of nicotine, heart disease, diabetes, high blood pressure…and diagnosed with calcific bursitis in her right shoulder last year. No significant family history. No further pain here…physical exam and EKG unremarkable…I'm thinking of sending her out with an anti-inflammatory, tell her to use heat, and schedule a follow-up appointment with her family physician in a few days."

"Where exactly was the pain?"

"Right upper back."

"Sore to the touch?"

"No."

"What else could it be—especially with shortness of breath and lightheadedness?"

"Well…except for the pain being on the right, the symptoms are consistent with angina…and if it was from her bursitis, it would make more sense for her shoulder to be tender when you push on it. But angina should be on the left, in the front of the chest."

"Does her body know that?"

"Excuse me?"

"Is there a law that says heart muscle deprived of blood flow will only send out its distress call on the port side of the vessel?"

"No."

"So what is it until proven otherwise?"

"Angina, unstable type, because the pain came on at rest when the heart wasn't being stressed. Which is a more ominous sign. And if we miss that, it could kill her."

"Tell the lucky lady she just bought herself a ticket to our world-class CCU."

He was right. The front wall of Mrs. Shaughnessy's left ventricle was teetering. With her chest cracked open to get at her heart, coronary bypass surgery extended her lease as one of the transients we all are in this life, and that was good. She wasn't ready to go.

All this, from Charlie, long before the major medical establishment stepped up to the plate and racked up a season of research, much of it done by female physicians pitching repeatedly to women and their bodies, and the big managers came to "realize" that this gender can present with "atypical" heart disease.

And when it's missed—it can kill them.

Breasts may be easier to check. Just before the turn of the last century Dr. William Halstead became famous for the radical mastectomy operation he designed in 1889 and that bears his name. He brought thoroughness and art to the discipline of surgery, making it more than just speed. But his namesake was a mutilating procedure, slicing off the entire mammary gland and the muscle and tissue behind it, all right to the bone, as well as the lymph glands connected to that area of the body and the arm on the same side. Even with appropriate clinical distance, as a medical student I found it a difficult undertaking to observe. In the manner of his time, and his peers, Halstead saw breast cancer as a surgically curable disease. He preached that this advance would not only cut off the tumor's blood supply but also sever its hold on human life. Over time, his design was "modified," but both men and women have continued to live in fear of the diagnosis he worked to conquer.

Breast cancer rightly—**RIGHTLY**—garners the money and focus it now commands. That diagnosis is a live grenade thrown at you and all who love you. But the loss of that pump within, and the rhythm of its swing, due to a choke hold on the red cells that ferry its oxygen life-support, has historically stolen more life from more women every year than the loss of a breast. Charlie, being slightly older than I, had assisted in the operating room at more radical mastectomies. He never picked apart a case presentation by a woman resident any differently than the way he carried out a formal dissection on one of the guys. He leaned gently on us all, leveraged by intelligence (and not everyone was as even-handed as that). I watched him deliver babies and remind us that women taught us how to bring a child into the world because they had been doing it a lot longer than doctors, especially male ones. And he was ahead of his time in seeing women patients as whole, with hearts that needed care.

Two weeks after my brush with near-disaster on Mrs. Shaughnessy, my first-year resident compatriots and I were huddled around Charlie at morning report (and I do mean morning, as in 6 am— you came in in the dark, and you went home in the dark; even when it was daylight savings time, they didn't save any daylight for you.). Harry Vaughn was presenting a patient he had admitted overnight. He'd gone through the history of the present illness, past medical history, habits (smoking, drinking, et al), allergies, meds, surgical history, family history, and review of systems (complaints in any of the body's organs and interacting departments, including skin). He gave us the physical exam findings, starting with the vital signs, and ending with the lab and other test results. He began his assessment of Mr. Belotti's diagnoses. I was trying not to fall asleep like I had talking on the phone last night to my college roommate.

"Number one. He's been excessively fatigued, and it's probably due to his anemia. Number two. He's been suffering from diffuse joint pains, which are most likely caused by his—"

"Stop." Charlie donned his Cheshire Cat smile. "Let's just go back to the differential diagnosis of fatigue."

"Can't I just do it my way?"

Another feces-eating grin. "Sure. But the polls are closed. We're not taking a vote today, so I'm still Moses."

Even Harry laughed. "Okay. The possible causes of anemia, in a male"—

"Thank you. I'm pleased that you've noted Mr. Belotti's primary and secondary sex characteristics, but I want you to think more globally."

"Why?"

"Stay with me on this, Harry. Believe it or not, I have a plan. One that has been passed down to me. And I'm on your side."

"Right. Well, the possible causes of fatigue—IN HUMANS—are anemia, cardiac, lung dysfunction, infection, chronic disease—"

"Which ones in particular?"

Harry twitched his right upper lip. "Ahh...kidney problems...diabetes..."

"Remember the basics you perform when you first meet a patient: inspection, palpation..."

"You want me to tell you how he looked?" Charlie nodded. "Cripes, whadda ya think? He looked tired!"

"Harry." A pause gentle to the air. "This is about what *you* think. It's not to harass you. Really."

Charlie spread his hands and scanned our group. "Ladies and gentleman, for twenty-five thousand dollars—maybe—and one extra night off call—impossible, the possible answers are..."

And we were off.

"Mr. Belotti could look puffy and be tired from an underactive thyroid gland causing fluid retention, but with anemia, say..."

"With anemia, due to occult GI bleeding from a silent ulcer, especially since he admits to at least four drinks a day, or a slow leak lower down from colon cancer, then he'd look pale, and depending on how low his blood count was, even that telltale lousy looking sallow color..."

"And as a long-term smoker, with some emphysema, he could be working harder to breathe, using accessory muscles of respiration, which would be clearly visible, and be a little cyanotic, a blue bloater, but on the other hand he could be plethoric, ruddy of face, because his body is manufacturing extra red cells to carry more oxygen per heartbeat in order to compensate for the decreased air exchange across scarred lung cell membranes, and this condition, called secondary polycythemia, would actually be manifested by a higher hematocrit, the opposite of anemia..." (This last aria coming from Jeff Madison, who could spin out more medical information with one inhalation than a diva at the

Metropolitan Opera, and someone whose brain, we laid bets, hurt at night…)

"But maybe the fatigue is from depression, and we need to know what's going on in the rest of his life, and that's why the hematocrit result doesn't show that much of an anemia…."

Charlie was like the new basketball coach who comes in and tells the team we're just going to run in practice and learn excellent defense, and it will all work out. We will be the best.

We stopped to catch our collective brain breaths and Charlie blew his whistle.

"And what if Mr. Belotti has all these things as the cause of his fatigue? Or two or three of them?"

"At the same time?" Jeff asked. He looked on the verge of cardiac arrest.

"Why not? Anything in the rule book make that illegal?"

We dribbled that ball for a moment.

"But a low thyroid condition isn't common in middle-aged men," Harry said.

Charlie stuck his hands in the pockets of his starched white coat and leaned back. He surveyed his players. "Guys—what if Mr. Belotti's body didn't read *Harrison's Textbook of Medicine*?"

Ellie Pardon put her hand up. "You mean like Jeff has, and memorized every damn last page?"

Even Jeff laughed.

By the end of the case discussion, especially because the patient also "looked sick" (see Rule #2), we had working diagnoses that included the onset of rheumatoid arthritis and bone marrow production of red cell size and shape assaulted due to an unoffical new indoor-record whiskey consumption, although the joint pains could also be a manifestation of thyroid disease. As we were pushing our chairs in, Charlie started to hum a tune. I knew it from somewhere.

"Remember. '*Just start at the very beginning, a very good place to start…* '"

Julie Andrews. *Do Re Mi.* From *The Sound of Music.* How could he!

"Hey—listen to me. Truly. This is not to hurt your ears. Go out there today, and day after day, and do it the same way. No cheating."

Shortchange yourself; shortchange the patient. Which was even worse. Use everything you know—it really isn't all wrong, and sometimes you know more than you think you do. If you don't play by the rules, and something happens to that patient, I want you to never forgive yourself. Even if nobody ever catches your mistake.

Charlie Parrish, a physician whose lust to provide care for a man or a woman, to parse out the helpful and hurtful, the obvious and occult in another's medical and human condition and come to the aid of that fellow traveler, intercepted me at a crossroads in my career. He wanted us to see what *could* be. In clinic, he showed us how to explain our work to patients and reasonably screen for any condition that we could fight together. Prevention meant looking ahead with all our smarts and heart. "Healing" was the name of the game, and that meant being fully present with the patient, giving it your best shot, and included staying there whether someone was in the beginning of their life, or at the end. Charlie taught as naturally as he breathed, because he loved every aspect of the game. Life, medicine—it was all breath-giving when it was afoot. There was nothing better than being given the skills and the chance to play on center court; and every patient was the main event.

And anybody could pop up with anything.

Winning, in medicine, was simple: Think fast, look for all the angles, pass when you need to, and remember the patient and you are on the same team. The patients who have crossed my path since have much to thank him for; and so do I.

We all learn differently, and from many people, and the flow goes back and forth—parents and their children, professors and medical students, patients with doctors. Charlie showed one teacher can make a major difference. Pass it on.

When he left us at the end of our first year of training, he wanted to go where he could do two things he dearly loved: be a real family doctor in a small town, and ski. It was Maine who got him.

We always said...that year they won the state championship in medicine ball.

Rule #6
Remember Abigail Adams

"Does this look like what a woman looks like to you?"

I leaned over Beth's shoulder so I could see what she was pointing at on her desk.

"Only in cartoon land," I said.

"Who draws these things? A mutant?"

"Has to be a male one who wants to grow up and be a doctor."

"And went from the terrible twos directly to mid-life crisis—changing wives."

Beth was reviewing the old records of a patient she was picking up in her practice. She had flipped a page to a female physical form, and this is what she saw:

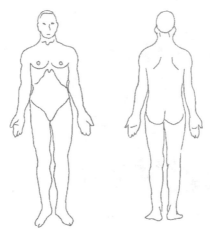

So—WHAT IS THIS? It can't be a mature man's vision of how God made Eve, because the hair and a few other angles are all wrong. (Or is that a hairnet seen from the back?) But absent the *membrum virile* and its two sidekicks, central items that Michelangelo was comfortable carving on his sculpture of David, it certainly isn't wholly male. (Unless...this illustration is unconsciously revealing how a rich doctor sees himself after the divorce settlement...)

In medicine you are encouraged to draw a picture when it adds to the clinical information you are trying to document; it clarifies the position of a wound, or the site of a rash, or the area where a breast mass is palpable. Hand-drawn attempts can be highly entertaining but poor facsimiles, making a sketch trying to show where the sutures have been put in a thumb laceration resemble an ill-advised sausage. Keeping things in proportion gets tricky even for clinicians with some artistic talent.

So it makes sense to standardize templates for common areas of examination, whether the body part is checked in the emergency room or at an office physical; and it's faster for doctors to complete when scrambling through paperwork. Just as in any kind of office, whether reading balance sheets or lab reports, people are more efficient in extracting important information if everyone gets used to seeing the same thing.

But over my years as a physician, I've seen some pictures that take some getting use to—and most of them are "depictions" of female anatomy. Here is a small gallery:

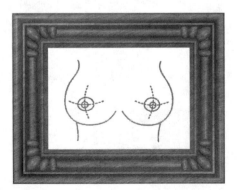

"The Tassels"
(aka "Sparkling Orbs")

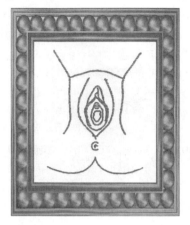

"The Scream"
(Perfectly named in the mind of many females, it is the sight a physician sees when he rolls his stool up to a woman in the pelvic exam position—and a chart visualization infrequently needed to doodle on, for it is rarely the site of the key gynecologic finding. It is akin to drawing a man's rear flanks in anticipation of a rectal and prostate exam. From that propective, calling it "The Scream" works for both genders.)

"Not Just Another Pretty Face"
(Nor a bashful one. It is a Picasso-like "Breasts and a Button In a Smiling Belly.")

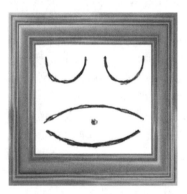

We "think" as we "see"—from a first impression on a date, to a fixed-view of race, to staring at another's religious adornment. Human brains need a sage "look-out" so that we do not unconsciously sideswipe each other. If a doctor "imagines" women in schoolboy-fashion, ill at ease with both himself and the totality of a female being, then he will think differently about a woman when she comes to him as a patient. And a truly "cock-eyed" picture will keep developing, blurring the shape of care.

I've often wondered what women patients would think if they saw these designs. Now I'll know.

I hope there wasn't some equally bizarre portrait of me in my chart at Dr. Stewart's office. Francis Xavier Stewart, MD, FACOG (Fellow of the American College of Obstetricians and Gynecologists—a fairly standard high-quality credential), FRCS (Fellow of the Royal College of Surgeons—expected in the British Isles, not common in this country, but can be acquired through exchange training and never fails to impress in the colonies), was the highest grosser in surgical billings at the hospital. I knew this on a numerical, factual basis, because a close friend of mine ran the accounts receivable department. Simply put, Francis X. Stewart brought in more money to the hospital than any other doctor because he admitted more patients in whom he removed something. This included babies.

He was also the "doctor's doctor," meaning that female physicians went to him, or colleagues sent the women in their lives to him. He knew how to cut—as expert with a scalpel in the operating room as he was in parting his Red Sea of acolytes at a medical staff meeting. In his office he had a framed drawing of rabbits in a conga dance, fading away into the distant perspective, entitled "Receding Hare Line"; but despite going bald, he retained the swagger and smile of the confidently good-looking. A man of the "Dr. Kildare" generation (a time when nurses stood up when the doctor entered the ward), who rose to become "King of the Hospital" on the hill. They say every woman falls in love with her obstetrician, (obviously another remnant of the time when "doctor" meant "male"), and Stewart's charm was unavoidable. He always told a woman with child that she looked beautiful, repeating what he said he told his wife with each of her six (Catholic before birth control) pregnancies. I experienced that firsthand when I became his patient for my third.

My first two children were delivered by a woman who had four children of her own. She was ten years older than I, only able to get an interview for her surgical residency program because her first name was a family name which was assumed to belong to a man. We shared stories of how much better, or not, the medical milieu was becoming for women. She told me if it came down to a choice between being with your sick child or an ill patient, find a colleague to see the patient—because you only have one mother, but there's always another doctor. She delivered both of my sons, working both times with crackerjack modern skills as well as a nurse from England who helped me ease the spine-snarling back labor with the first one by administering "therapeutic touch": the warmth of hands hovering, focused, just above the skin, combined with tandem breathing with your caregiver so that you believe that this pain, too, shall pass. But we moved in the time between child number two and number three, and I had to find another excellent physician. Sully was a tough act to follow.

I loved being pregnant, never had any complications, and didn't seem to have any morning or later in the day sickness—but maybe that was because my body knew I couldn't have that happen and miss work. It wasn't an option. Because I was the only woman in my medical group, one of my male colleagues had suggested that I "should have done extra night-call ahead" if I knew I was "going to do this." (I thought about reminding him of that when he had his heart attack a few years later, but I was too well brought up. Besides, my darling mother said "Leave him to God—He gets around to everybody.")

I also mimicked my mother with relatively short labors, getting quicker with each succeeding event, and for the last month of my pregnancy with my daughter I walked around halfway to splashdown at five centimeters of dilated cervix. I followed all of Dr. Stewart's recommendations to the letter, except for the one about not traveling more than ten miles from the hospital because of my brisk births. Two weeks before my due date I eloped over state lines to my 20th Brown undergraduate reunion: I was confident both in the expertise of the physicians who had trained me in medical school on the OB-GYN rotation and that I remembered exactly how to get to Women and Infants Hospital from my alma mater (the "bounteous mother" of us all). Besides, I knew how to deliver a baby—and I could coach my husband if need be in the car. I figured the stars of medicine were with me.

My two sons were born on their due dates, almost exactly nine months to the hour from the time of conception. But my daughter was her own woman, and I spent five extra days of a record hot June waiting for her. I went into the hospital on the sixth with a plan that I would be induced if necessary.

That morning, Dr. Stewart checked me, chatted with my husband who worked in the hospital administration, and "artificially ruptured" my membranes.

"Hey Bill, nice tie," he said to my husband as they both stood at the bedside.

"Yeah, I like it, too. Phyllis got it for me for Christmas last year."

I was speechless because as soon as my water broke, I felt the elevator descend rapidly to the pelvic floor, and the doors were about to open.

"I have to push!"

The team went into action. I only had to push twice, and out came the sweetheart who had somersaulted in my womb.

Two days later, Francis Stewart gave me a kiss on the cheek, pronounced both my baby daughter and me beautiful, and set us free. I went back for my six-week postpartum check, and two weeks later the telephone rang as I was nursing my real live doll.

"Is this Phyllis?...Phyllis, this is Sylvia, in Dr. Stewart's office. Your PAP smear is abnormal, and you have to come back for some more tests."

I didn't know Sylvia, among the legions of handmaidens in one of the busiest practices in the city; and since she hadn't addressed me as "Doctor," I presumed she didn't know what I did for a living. I let it go that it hadn't been a colleague-to-colleague call. So was that all the explanation a "regular" patient got? I knew the levels of microscopic abnormality in PAP smears, and the probable next-step protocols—but I had had twenty years of normal yearly smears. Even I was dumbfounded, and worried. What about the other poor lay souls that Sylvia "touch-toned?"

I had a repeat PAP smear, a sampling of the junction of the cervix and uterine neck, and a biopsy of the lining of the womb.

The second PAP still had abnormal cells, some "possibly" precancerous, so I was moved along to removal of a circumferential section of the cervix, a "cone biopsy," under general anesthesia, to determine the geography of the renegade cells. I awoke from the anesthesia (administered by a fellow physician of whom I had to ask his name) with no memory, just "lost time," trying not to think about the less-than-decent way I'd sometimes seen unconscious women put in the pelvic exam position in the operating room. My throat hurt from the endotracheal "breathing" tube, and I bled, with clots, for two weeks—when I called, thinking I shouldn't just try to treat myself, I got Sylvia. I returned to my initial thought.

At the end of a day in the office filled with emergency add-ons of patients with bronchitis or stomach flu, and children, sweet smiling but nonetheless with streams of runny nose to varying degree and trajectory, I started to feel the muscle aches (like an eighteen-wheeler had ironed me) and starting fever of a flu syndrome. I had just returned to work from a short maternity leave, and I wanted to go home to see my baby, have her empty my bulging breasts, and go to bed. My nurse came to the door of my office.

"Dr. Stewart's on the phone for you."

"Phyllis. Your biopsy shows the precancerous cells may be through several layers. You need a hysterectomy."

It didn't matter how Mr. OB-GYN was acting, or my advanced degree; I already felt in the role of the patient. We'd studied the body of literature on that at Brown, so we could vicariously put ourselves in those shoes as physicians. I was vulnerable, and somewhat dependent. I felt slapped when I was down.

"I can't. There must be some other option. You know we were considering having one more child." I knew tears were breaking through, and he could hear them in my voice.

"Make an appointment to see me in the office."

I went home to tell my husband, but Francis had already broken confidentiality and called him. "She's acting hysterical. See if you can talk some sense into her. She should know better as a doctor."

Hysterical. Not according to the definition taught to us by our psychiatry professors, not by my reckoning. But an easy term to scatter around. Hysterical—did he even get the joke considering the operation he was recommending?

Two weeks went by. Knowing this particular cervical beast was slow-growing, I told my husband I'd rather take my chances on how quickly any microscopic changes would progress to full-blown carcinoma eating through its cage. I'd rather that than go back to Stewart in the OR, especially in a Proustian way. None of it felt right.

Still, I scrambled to find the right person for a second opinion. I needed Boston, someone outside my local sphere, where Stewart was untouchable. A physician friend in our multi-specialty group got me a name from a woman who had trained with a Dr. Conti, and said he was "different." Sure. Gynecologists train as surgical subspecialists—why would he want to conserve my body tissue?

Richard Conti took my cold call. He listened to the case.

"The literature on that subject is written by a bunch of old farts. A hysterectomy is a big deal. It's an amputation."

I was his.

He and his pathologists re-examined my cone biopsy slides—the "precancer" was only superficial, and not as severe as advertised. With a spinal anesthetic, I underwent the directly visualized laser removal of only the abnormal areas, (not the "blind sweep" I'd had), which was a procedure I had researched and read was then being done at teaching centers. Everyone in the outpatient surgery center associated with my case introduced themselves. The head of anesthesia (he didn't tell me he was) saw me sitting on a gurney, waiting my turn and reading, and asked if I wanted a little more privacy and pulled the curtain around my stretcher.

But besides my doctor, the one person I will never forget was the young lady who checked me in. It was December and I was shivering a little, and probably not just from the cold. She smiled at me and these were her first words: "Would you like a heated blanket?" From the support personnel to the Harvard

Medical School-affiliated "big shots," everyone liked and understood his or her job: to serve another human being who asks for help. Without waiting to be asked.

I confronted Francis Stewart, but even for me as a colleague it was unnerving. It did not concern him that he had omitted discussing the laser alternative with me; he would not address whether he was familiar with it. I left his office thinking he put all those kids through private school by "virtue" of the women who hadn't stood up to him, or gotten a second opinion, because of his personal power. All that money from all those women on their backs.

So what of all the patients who tell physicians "I had a terrible experience with a doctor"? What about the ones whom a family member has to drag in, or can't, when they need us, because of "No more goddamn doctors!" I was on my way to being one of those patients, even though I believe in my craft. Each of us must realize we are critical to restoring their faith. It is the incontrovertible way we need to work with at least a glimmer of joy, even on a tough day, at being given the chance to do so, and watch that tiny brightness often become large light once a doctor and a patient start to move toward each other.

We may be a conduit of grace put here. We are blessed as physicians to offer small balm.

Women carry much with them. They may not run the world nor be fully recognized in some religions, but they are often blamed for much that goes wrong. "She asked for it"—the lady wore a tight skirt and got raped, the wife nagged her husband so he hit her. "This kid's going to prison"—well, she's a single mother. "She's just another pregnant teenager"—she should have practiced abstinence. (I particularly like that one, proving that my medical education was incorrect. Sperm are products of spontaneous generation and then swim through air. And it doesn't take two to tango.)

Overweight women come to my office who have put off a physical for years because they were embarrassed by another doctor. They felt they were seen as "just blobs." Unfortunately that physician is often male—and I can't help but ask if he looks like an anorexic. (Cardiologists like this are especially interesting—setting perhaps a little too intense an example?). Who are we to judge? These women already feel lousy about how their health is affected by their weight, about how the world sees them; their self-esteem has been flushed out to sea. It often is truly "there but for the grace of God" for us, because of our parents, our brains, our opportunities. They want to take better care of themselves, and we must encourage and explain how to do that. But these women are the caregivers, often of multiple generations. Their stress can be relentless. I once had a patient undergoing chemotherapy treatment for breast cancer, and she was taking care of her mother-in-law because her husband "wouldn't do it." She had to climb a flight of stairs to bring trays of food to this woman, balancing them with one arm that was swollen like an elephant's leg due to the loss of the lymph glands on that side (glands that drain and "recirculate" excess tissue fluid)—because of a Halstead radical mastectomy. More heartbreaking, in the hospital her surgeon refused to order "Reach to Recovery" visits so fellow victims of breast cancer could comfort her and give her life's hope.

I've seen women who have complained of being "tired all the time," and never had thyroid tests done because "that's not needed—you're just depressed." Where does control "profit" you as a physician? At least check the damn organ system—why not? The tests are not expensive and thyroid problems are more common in women. Imagine how you'd feel all day, every microscopic minute of every function, if your "master gland" wasn't working up to speed, affecting all body processes from skin turnover rates to heart rate to lipid profiles to the amount of flow and frequency of periods—and all these with secondary effects. All this making it a mythic struggle, ever harder, to take care of your family, your job. Yourself. And the person you go to for their help doesn't do what he can. What do you think—depressed yet?

Remember these women—absolutely—can have more than one thing going on at a time. Yes, they may "hate their miserable life," but despite their best efforts they may be financially imprisoned, especially if there are children—and with a spouse who has been brought up in a home, a culture, a religion, where women aren't equally valued. Who picks on his wife because she's "gotten fat." When these guys do come in I see the striking lack of perfection in their bodies and I am ready to ask with kindred bluntness: "Do you have a mirror, sir? Do your eyes work?"

A thirty-eight-year-old woman comes to see me repeatedly for depression and irritability.

"My husband says I'm hell to live with. You gotta do something. And I have no sex drive."

We go through endocrine and other indicated questions about symptoms, and I order thyroid among other tests. She comes back.

"All your results are normal."

"So why am I so tired?"

"What's your typical day like?"

She thinks for a moment. "I get up at five, make breakfast and lunches, drop the kids off at school on my way to work. I work in the meat department at the Big Deal Market, in and out of the freezer all day. Go home, make dinner, pick up the house a little and do laundry."

"What does your husband do?"

"He goes to work—he does construction—and he helps with the kids. Gives them their baths." She smiles. "They're six and eight."

"How's your marriage?"

"Oh great, you know. We started dating in high school. I mean—we're fine. I still love him. He's upset I don't want to have sex, and I know I'm not that attractive anymore, and he's gained a little weight, but I don't have time to exercise. I mean, maybe that would give me more energy. I should do that."

"Ever felt depressed before? Any family history?"

"I don't know. Not anything big. Never thought about killing myself. Maybe my mother was depressed." She stopped. "She was always worn out."

Linda wants to try Zoloft because her friend "felt better on it," even though I tell her it might make her lack of libido worse. She comes back after two weeks.

"Boy, I feel better. My husband says so, too. Says I'm nicer to be around. But you were right—the sex problem is worse. My husband's pretty frustrated, and I feel bad for him."

We switch to Wellbutrin. She has no sexual side effects, but she fees irritable again. And still tired. And still no interest in making love with her husband.

"How do you feel when you get home at night?"

"Exhausted."

"Do you think anybody would be that interested in sex if they're that tired?"

"No."

"So tell your husband. Tell him you'll feel more like making love if he does more around the house."

She wants to stay on the Wellbutrin because she thinks "it helps a little." She makes another follow-up appointment.

"Things are a little better. Ron is trying to help. But I still get angry for no reason."

"About what kind of things?"

Linda chews on her lip. "Well, about Ron, I guess. He likes to eat sunflower seeds, and he leaves the shells all over the house." I wait. "And he drives my van and I have to clean them all up from there, too."

"You've told him this makes you crazy?"

"Yeah—but nothing changes."

I could smell the nidus of the irritation.

"Okay," I say. "What group of humans makes a mess all over the place, doesn't want to clean up after themselves, and always wants something from Mom?"

She smiles. "Kids."

"Tell Ron you love him, he's a great guy, but when you're angry at him you get irritable and you're not interested in making love. And you don't want to have sex with a child."

We taper her off the antidepressant. Linda says she'll put her foot down.

I walk in the door at her next visit. New woman. Big smile. No drugs.

"Ron and I are both happy."

Put yourself in the position of these women. Literally. Progressive medical schools have the male students undress from the waist down, put a sheet over what's naked, and slide down to the end of the exam table with their feet in the stirrups: the "lithotomy position." They won't forget it. (And although I empathize with men who have to undergo a rectal/prostate exam, remember women also get that as part of their physicals. It's two to one). It is a posture and acrobatic maneuver necessary to accomplish in order to undergo a complete gynecologic check, because the designer of humans wisely put the organs that bring forth the continuation of the species into a well-protected place. But it is an "invasive procedure" also—it is not just cardiac catheterizations where a foreign object enters near the groin. And it may be the stupidest position in the world, making a person completely vulnerable, and if there was a fire alarm the poor soul in that contortion would be the last to get out because she could break her ankle trying to rapidly extricate her feet.

The role of women in medicine has improved. Elizabeth Blackwell became the first woman physician in the United States in 1849, graduating at the head of her class from Geneva Medical School in New York. Because she had faced rejection from all the other schools in her quest, along with founding The New York Infirmary for Women and Children she went on to establish Geneva Woman's Medical College. Women were allowed to enter Johns Hopkins Medical School only because its founding, in 1893, was made possible by a lavish gift from Mary Elizabeth Garrett—one of the key stipulations mandating that women be admitted to the school on equal terms with men and "enjoy all its advantages on the same terms as men." But Abraham Flexner's Report in 1910, commissioned by the American Medical Association and a landmark in setting quality and social responsibility goals for medical education in this country and Canada, was a factor in closing minority and women-only programs, saying they didn't fit "the standard."

My entering medical school class at Brown in 1973 had twenty women out of sixty students—ahead of its time. Women members of the profession are increasing, but not in numbers of academic promotions or as department heads. Women in charge of medical schools would, I believe, bring a different conversation to the table of power, just as women patients do. Clinical teaching, which women often excel at, is not considered as important in tenure decisions. A doctor can make more money doing more men's care, for doing a prostate biopsy is reimbursed by insurance companies at a higher price than taking a sample of the uterine lining. But research continues to show that there is still not income parity, even when men and women work the same hours in the same specialty.

As the dean of a medical school, I would look for a certain keen breed of candidate. The admission criteria would change: Those who seek medicine, to understand humanity, as naturally and critically as breathing, and have both the brain power and brain balance to sustain that quest, reveling, would go to the head of the class. The culture of medicine could then change, as it needs to, so that so many patients would not still complain of impersonal "care." Patients often tell women physicians more of what's on their mind; but they also do this with male physicians who lay out a bigger welcome mat. A male executive can see a physician and rave about him—but sadly, the poll results may be very different among that doctor's female patients. Is that a "great" doctor?

Male obstetrician/gynecologist; male obstetrician/gynecologist. Just let that bang back and forth in your head. It doesn't have to be an oxymoron. In the 1950s women in labor were put into "twilight sleep," so they didn't have to witness the birth of their babies. My mother went in to the hospital (with her efficient labor), and the doctor told her, "You'll have your baby in five minutes!"—but she wasn't awake to see me enter the world. What a vital event to steal from a woman. (At one point later in my life, as a physician, if I had run into that guy I might have slugged him). In the 1960s to 1970s, hysterectomy with or without the removal of the fallopian tubes and ovaries was the most commonly performed surgical procedure in this country. At the same time, Valium was the leader in drug prescriptions, primarily written by OB/GYNs—"mother's little helper," immortalized in a Rolling Stones song. For years, when taking a history I asked women what was the indication for their hysterectomies (cancer/true precancer dictating different follow-up), and many didn't know—nor have any idea how much of their tissue was taken. Some would cry, still mourning a visceral loss, different but akin to a miscarriage and how these were insensitively treated in the past.

I took care of a woman who had "avoided" an equivocally indicated hysterectomy because she wanted "to go out of this world with everything I came in with." She wondered if the reason "those doctors" sometimes took out both the uterus and the tubes and ovaries was because "they got paid by the pound." (They do weigh surgically removed organs in the pathology lab, but not to up the fee).

Remember, as my own career experience and adventures as a patient so deeply show, it is not the gender of the physician that counts—it is the degree of jerkdom. We owe it our patients to not act like disinterested (and often uninteresting) jerks, and our profession needs to see this problem and address it. Too many patients, especially women, the group that goes to the doctor more often (for physiological reasons, and less-stubborn-than-men reasons, and, dare I say, braver reasons), still feel let down.

Hidden black holes in the mind of a doctor affect outcomes—and how soon the diagnosis gets to come out. At a point in my career when I had had time to polish the "brass accoutrements" which years earlier a supportive surgeon had told me I'd need as the only woman on our medical staff, another male colleague stepped on a land mine of his own making. We were both senior physicians. At a meeting of the department he chaired, with about fifty both support and provider staff present, Dr. Hadley proudly announced that I, two other women clinicians, and the three thousand female patients we took care of were joining his team. He then victoriously proclaimed this meant "my department now has the most vaginas." I was delayed finishing with a patient that day, and missed his performance—but I am not making this up, because two young and very decent male nurses were so uncomfortable with his words they came to tell me.

A firestorm ensued, initiated by others. I watched and then one day went to Hadley's office and stood at his door, smiling.

"Were you drunk?"

"No…" His chair squeaked.

"You're lucky I wasn't there."

"Yes, I know, I should have…"

I smiled a little more. "I would have knocked your teeth down your throat."

(The proper use of that last phrase was taught to me by a young male physician when I was a department head. He was as good a clinician and human being as he had been a college hockey star. He slid into my office one day to complain about a slightly older woman doctor who consistently annoyed all of us and noted "that if she was a man I'd take her out back and knock her teeth down her throat." Slap shot right on target. Nothing like it.)

Dr. Hadley apologized and then stealth apologized to the entire office on email, and then apologized to me, unsolicited, for several months whenever he saw me. I said, "Let it go." Six months later, as part of his teaching position, he became the overseer of stress testing for our patients. I sent him a woman with atypical chest pain, and noted I was concerned she had underlying cardiac disease.

"I don't think a stress test is warranted in this patient, as her symptoms are not classic for heart disease," came back in reply to my request for consultation. Think about this; see previous chapter. Think about this again—he was *teaching* young physicians.

Now think, especially, about this because it affects someone's life. Someone's medical care. A fellow human being's care. The patient was as aghast and ill-served as I was (maybe more, considering her previous medical experiences a la "I told you what I told you"). I had to send her out of our system, and you can guess the end of the story. That doctor, a well-adjusted man, was happy to clinch the diagnosis. So it is vital—*critical to care*—that physicians practice by "the rules"—and know themselves, especially their own biases.

Finally—remember Abigail Adams. The wife of John Adams, he the second President of the United States and a delegate to the Constitutional Convention in 1789. Abigail and John's voluminous correspondence reveals the high intelligence and deep mutual respect of each—especially from John to Abigail. Often alone, she skillfully managed a farm, a budget (at times very lean), and their children, as John traveled long distances and was away for long periods of time doing his equally vital work.

Abigail wrote John: "Remember the ladies." She did not live to see that incorporated into the Constitution of our country—but as physicians, we can incorporate that value into our own "constitutions": the conditions of our minds, our dispositions, our temperaments. Manifest it in what constitutes our character—our fundamental principles.

What we are made of will make our profession, our work for others, that which can stand the test of time.

Rule #7
'Til Death Do Us Part

"I think I need to make an appointment."

It was the week before Christmas, and the end of the workday. Anne Cheresh was on the phone with me, polite and understated as always. Too much so.

"I've got this pain in my epigastric area, can't seem to get rid of it. My blood count, liver tests are normal, there's no nausea, vomiting, diarrhea, blood in the stool—but it isn't responding to any of the meds."

"Ever have this before?"

"No, not exactly. They thought I might have had an ulcer when I was in school, but it went away with Tums and Zantac. I don't even put it down when I fill out past medical history forms." Silence; then a pulled-in breath. "And besides, things are going great. I'm having the time of my life."

"What's the pain feel like?"

"Constant gnawing. Even when I eat something."

"Losing weight? Feel full too fast?"

"I don't think so. Maybe a little."

"Any new bad habits?"

She laughed. "No. No booze or cigarettes."

"You did all these tests on yourself, right?"

"Of course," said Dr. Anne Cheresh. "You know me—I didn't want to overreact."

No kidding. I'd met Anne when she was a second-year family medicine resident in a program where I was the associate director. We were only separated in age by five years, for Anne had gone to medical school late after teaching chemistry. Married and ready to start a family, she suffered serial miscarriages instead, it finally becoming clear that she was unable to carry a child to term because her mother had been given a then-popular hormone to prevent premature labor when she was pregnant with Anne. The irony was not lost on her; but the sadness in her womb never strayed to her lips or her face.

But her husband did stray. His paramour called Anne at our clinic to announce her pregnancy. Anne swallowed that, denying any heartburn, and proceeded to end the marriage as methodically as she did her charts. She finished her training, traveled to Africa and China, and came back to join a multi-specialty group where I now was. This year I'd seen her for her physical, when she broke her right wrist on an Outward Bound cruise—and as a colleague at meetings.

Her appointment was at two-thirty the next afternoon. When I opened the exam room door and saw her, I knew one thing immediately: she's dying. I heard those words in my mind as surely as if someone was reading them to me. Anne's weight was down more than "a little." She looked fragile, the muscles of the woman who had climbed rigging on a tilting sailboat only a prior picture.

"Anne. Did you eat anything today, yesterday…last week?"

Her gaze wobbled. "I haven't been that hungry."

I carefully palpated the area over the pit of her stomach, and she winced. I thought I felt a mass through her abdominal wall. I set up GI films for the next day.

The chief radiologist interrupted my ten o'clock well-child check.

"The stinking thing is taking up 95 percent of the inside of her stomach. It's a miracle she isn't obstructed. We'll need Matt Kulik to stick a scope down and biopsy it for tissue diagnosis, but it's got to be cancer." Quiet. "Jesus."

Anne wasn't obstructed because she was barely putting anything down her food tube. The stomach cancer was hijacking the few calories coming in, stuffing them into its terrorist cells. The rest of Anne was starving. And she knew it; she'd known. The pain had been constant for four months, not the two she'd told me initially. She knew exactly how much weight she'd lost. She didn't "want to make a fuss about it" because she didn't want to lose hold of the life she'd just gotten back. She didn't want to tell her brother, her only relative, or the man who was in love with her now.

Joseph Caldemone was the surgeon who knifed out as much of the tumor as he could without leaving her with no gut. Anne had done a rotation with him as a medical student, assisted him in the same operating room where he opened her up, and his heart was broken at her now gaunt smile. Anne left the hospital and the oncologist offered her the triple drug regimen of chemotherapy poison, which we all knew had a rotten reputation—but it was all we had.

"What do you think?" Anne was sitting in the exam room with me, bulked up in a thick sweater disguise. "What should I say?"

"About the chemo?"

"No." She was smiling. "Tomorrow's New Year's Eve. What should I say if an old friend calls me up? 'Happy New Year! I'm dying!'"

"Did you tell your brother yet?"

"No. It'll kill him."

"Very funny. Look—he's divorced, your parents are dead. You and he are the last of the Mohicans. I'll call him if you want me to."

"No. I'll do it." She leaned forward. "But what would you do about the chemo?"

"You're young, you're a stubborn pain in the ass—I guess I'd have to try it once. It's only a 5 percent success rate, but somebody's got to be in that sliver."

She was in the third week of treatment when I saw her again. Her lungs were clear, she was holding steady on her weight with high-powered nutrition drinks, and her blood tests were good. She'd seen Caldemone for a post-op check the week prior to seeing me.

"He saw this?" I asked. I was palpating where the body's head-to-toe internal chain of lymph glands surfaced with evidence: at the neck, groin, armpit, and above the clavicle. Tender lymph nodes in the first three places were good, showing the body was responding to a possible infection; but a nontender lump in the fourth area was a lousy sign for traveling malignancy. And that was exactly where Anne now had one that was feeling no pain as it leaned on the bone—along with a new swelling hogging the incision line on her abdomen. That was where my hands stopped. But neither mass was sitting pretty.

Anne looked up at me from her prone position on the table. "Yes, Dr. Caldemone, God, I still call him that—Joe—saw it. He said it was just a fluid collection around the suture site."

I kept my hand over the soft bulge in her skin and my eyes on her face. "What do you think?"

"I think it's the cancer thumbing its nose in the face of the chemo. And he couldn't tell me."

Anne refused the second course of chemo. She'd given the drugs their chance at fame. She worked half days, seeing people who weren't acutely infectious, for as long as she could, tormenting the rest of us in the ladies room by noting that her wig never had a bad hair day. She came in to see me for a resizing of her diaphragm as she lost weight, so that as she lingered on life's joys to the end, on the timeless comfort of skin to skin, there would be no more "almost" children to mourn. Then she went home: where she could play her mother's baby grand piano, talk to her brother Edward, be held by her love, Patrick—and die.

Two days before she did I made a house call. I sat on the side of her bed, holding her hand. She'd deep-sixed the wig. When the hospice nurse went downstairs to make coffee, Anne opened her eyes.

"My parents fought all the time. We lived in Paris for a while because of my father's work, we had a summer house in Maine—but I always thought booze and money were the only things that kept my mother and father going. They both died as alcoholics." She kept her eyes fixed on mine. "Edward and I learned to be very, very quiet. He got loud later. But I never did."

She tried to squeeze my hand. "That's what killed me. I swallowed everything, I was always nice. Always. I kept every-thing in—and it ate me up." She smiled her old smile. "I waited too long to scream."

I had a patient who wore this tee shirt to his appointments: *"Eat right. Exercise. Die anyway."* He'd come in and tease me that trying to do the right thing and be healthy was ever more hopeless because "you medical people keep changing what's good for us." But both he and Anne knew that every day above ground is a gift, because everybody gets something. Live like mad as long as you can; even with cancer, you're alive each day until you die. If you are the doctor taking care of that patient, if you also give her the best you've got, it is no failure when she dies. You never pos-sessed the final power over dust to dust.

As physicians and patients, we each step along the human line between life and death with every heartbeat. Here one moment—gone the next. When doctors can't deal with death, can't talk to a patient and his family about a life's end, *then* they have failed. They have failed at their sworn duty to the patient to be a physician until death do us part. Their silence—their avoidance—broadcasts to all what they have turned their backs on.

If you'd come into the world in 1914 with my mother, you couldn't have done that. Her mother gave birth to most of her eleven children at home, and they all attended Uncle Jamie's wake in another house, watching (and singing) "out the window he must go, he must go, he must go" when his casket wedged itself tight coming through the front door. In their Irish music they saw death as crazy-continuous with life:

"When a guy dies that's the best fun of all,
　We pitches in and we hires a hall;
　We gets a bathtub and fills it with gin,
　Then we throw the poor sucker right in—
　And dead or alive, you should see that bum swim!"

But now so many doctors are nowhere near as comfortable with death, and just can't wait to do a little jig with the dying patient and his family, and then change partners—moving to someone who won't ask uncomfortable questions when in the arms of another. This is the physician who can't say directly to an eighty-five-year-old woman or her family that the reason she shouldn't continue to live alone is that she could fall and die alone. In our techno-medicine country, it is epitomized by the radiation oncologist my uncle saw for his inoperable lung cancer, the doctor who degreed the parameters of the "last hurrah" treatment to bomb his insurgent tumor and keep an oxygen highway open to one side of his chest. I spoke to her about his advance directive, and she couldn't wait to tell me she was "only in charge of his radiation therapy" even as I was calling to tell her that if he stopped breathing in *her* department, under one of *her* machines, we wanted *her* to know *his* resuscitation request.

In her eighty-fourth year, my mother was completely submerged by Alzheimer's Disease. She was living with my family, first occasionally getting lost driving the children back from a soccer practice. She began to dote on the cats, a species she had despised ever since one had peed in a new pair of shoes (she was the Imelda Marcos of Boston)—she let them in and out in a repetitive audio and video loop forgetting that "poor kitty" had been in and out ten times in fifteen minutes. When a week went by without her sitting down at our Wurlitzer organ to play her daily medley of *Oklahoma* show tunes that culminated in "Take Me Out To The Ballgame," I knew she was no longer herself. Phyllis Catherine Hollenbeck was a trained musician, had perfect pitch, and could play by ear; now she couldn't play by brain. And the other kick to the head was that she was only on eye drops for glaucoma and could hike at a mall as fast as my fifteen-year-old son.

The idea of history, including September 11, 2001, ceased to exist for her. For a while she tried to "walk home to Boston" from the opposite coast every night, readying herself for the trip by taking a plastic bag out of a wastebasket and packing her gold slippers in it. As she lost all memory of her marriage to a man "like no other," the "rare bird," Protestant variety, who wooed her with Roger and Hammerstein's "People Will Say We're In Love," she also relinquished the idea of a mother who took her to see Babe Ruth at Fenway Park. Knowledge of her children and grandchildren, her brothers and sisters, of all the reality of her life, tapered off, as did the ability to feed, clean, and know to dress herself. I cared for her at my house for two years, then felt pushed to break a promise to myself: I must place her in a nursing home because I had to return to full-time work. Thank God by that point my mother no longer knew there was a word for "home."

She suffered one bout of aspiration pneumonia because she inhaled some soup while trying to swallow it, the small door directing solids and water to the esophagus and away from the trachea unable to swing as trained without further instruction from her atrophied brain. I agreed with the doctor about treating her with antibiotics, but that if it happened again we would again discuss what to do. She rallied, a year went by, but her body's sense of coordination of the mechanism of swallowing became more and more of a fantasy. And then the sound of her voice disappeared as phonation and articulation vanished from her repertoire of skills. The witty conversationalist, my unconditional champion and friend—silent.

My mother and I had talked multiple times over the years about her wishes regarding extraordinary and artificial means of life support, and a duly witnessed and notarized paper to that extent was in her chart at the nursing home. She wanted little. As a Roman Catholic from her bone marrow, she said, "I've been aiming for heaven all my life." She saw no need to argue with God when she got the call.

I was seeing patients on a Wednesday when one of the young women covering our phones told me there was a call from

Evangeline, the registered nurse at my mother's nursing home. Susan hadn't thought she should just take a message.

"Doctor Hollenbeck, your mother can't swallow her pills."

"What pills?"

"The antibiotics."

"What antibiotics?"

"The ones for her pneumonia."

This was getting ridiculous. And this was the first I'd heard about her second diagnosis of aspiration pneumonia. She'd spiked a fever late that morning after breathing in whatever bits of her last dinner hadn't leaked onto her dress. Dr. Felix had not deigned to call me, but at least Evangeline had.

I tracked down Dr. Felix by the end of the day. This took determination, as it can be almost as difficult for two doctors to connect on the phone during working hours as it is for a patient calling to get through to their one doctor.

"What are you doing?" I asked.

"Well, the xray looks like probable early aspiration pneumonia, so of course I started treatment."

"What about her clearly spelled out wishes and our agreement?"

"I was sure you'd want her on meds. We can give the Augmentin IV if we have to."

"And she'll keep inhaling even water. Where are we going with this?"

"Well, I can order a speech therapy consult and they can help her learn to swallow again."

What? When did my mother and I buy admission tickets to Magic Medicine Land? "This isn't someone who's had a stroke," I said. "My mother doesn't have any viable cortex to retrain. It won't take."

I drove to see my mother and talked to Evangeline again.

"Hold the antibiotics in the morning. I don't want her choking on a pill."

I kissed my mother, went home, and prayed. I called her two remaining brothers in Boston.

"She'll need a feeding tube after this, even if she doesn't end up in the hospital with a complication of the pneumonia."

"Phyllis, we trust your judgement on this. You're the doctor," Uncle Gerard said. "But you know she's ready, and I believe this is a sign. It's okay to let her go."

When I was younger, even as a new mother, I couldn't imagine what I'd do without my own mother. "God isn't ready for me yet," she'd tell me. "Don't worry. Nothing's going to happen to me now because I've still got work to do." I studied the picture of her sitting on the floor with me one Christmas when I was two, the tree on top of the Philco television set in its cabinet. She'd gone on to help take care of all six of her grandchildren; she'd been my dependent for years according to the IRS as I took care of her. Things had come full circle, and it seemed clear it wasn't to be broken now. Not by those of us on earth, and not after a second message.

Still—while I was *a* doctor, I wasn't *the* doctor on this case. I was the daughter of a patient, struggling with the most Herculean decision of my existence. But between my work schedule and Felix's foot-dragging at calling me back after work, I hadn't been able to schedule a face-to-face meeting with him.

I called Evangeline the next day from my office.

"How's she doing?"

"Ready to smile at everyone, as ever. Only a little fever. Not really coughing, even though the radiologist confirmed it's right upper lobe pneumonia again."

"She wouldn't want more medicines, so I don't want her on any more antibiotics. I need Dr. Felix to change his orders."

"You could call hospice. They'll come here."

I did. They ran interference, and Felix fell away. I never saw him again. The hospice people also took care of me and my children. The plan was to let my mother dehydrate naturally as the small amounts of fluid she could get down dwindled away, and to give her a small dose of morphine if she became anxious in breathing, or otherwise. She never did. I knew this was a painless death, but only because I was a physician—*not* because of the patient's doctor guiding the path.

On the last Sunday of my mother's life, I sat alongside her on her bed, "watching" TV, our legs stretched out parallel to each other's and my arm around her shoulders. She sat staring at a place I didn't know, but occasionally I turned towards her and she seemed to smile. All at once it hit me she would be truly gone in a day or two, flesh and blood gone, even though I'd already lost her several years ago. The double death of Alzheimer's.

I slipped to my knees in the same posture I'd find her in at night when I was a child; she'd see me at the door with a question on my face, and with a nod, motion me in with one hand and leave the other one up in the air in the prayer stance. Now I leaned over her bed, my head on her knees, my fingers pressed together, and started to cry.

I felt her hand on my back, and she started to rub it slowly and gently, in circles. Just like when I was a child. I looked up and she smiled—comforting me as she said goodbye. Forty-eight hours later her soul was on its way.

The hospice volunteers described her as "grace-filled." To me, she also had perfect pitch in everything she did. I believe she would get a big kick out of knowing (as she probably does) that I am channeling her Irish sayings.

There are good deaths; I have seen them in my own family and with patients. Perhaps people die as they live. I also believe that physicians can try, and must try, to help those they take care of leave this existence with grace and peace. Even if this happens in the emergency room. Each time, each person is often unpredictably unique. Each needs to make peace with his or her own and ethical way. Remember—as doctors *we work for the patient*. That is our job, and it is paramount in those times (which are not uncommon) when the medical choices do not point to a perfect answer. We explain the options for heart disease treatment, for knee surgery, for diagnosing the cause of fever; we should not shirk this role of trust and honor at any other point in a human life. With our understanding of the body's mechanisms and the coping wish of the mind and heart, we must aid and guide others to "be not afraid" of caring for those who are dying—at home, if possible. A hospital death is to be avoided. It is often a solo passage: sudden, with family unable to make it in time, or prolonged, then all at once alone at two o'clock in the morning. Noticed only when the nurse comes to take vital signs. As a first year-resident I was called to pronounce an elderly man who had died that way. In the soulless fluorescent light left on above his bed I listened to his heart and checked his lungs; and then recognized a "scapular": two cloth rectangles, each with a piece of religious relic and linked by ribbon, which are put on over the head and lie front and back like tiny shields. His was green and white and twisted over his ribs. Instinctively I gave it back its rightful place—and then wondered who loved him enough to give it to him. And who wasn't there at that moment.

If a doctor is trained right, and the right kind of human being is picked for the job, neither life nor death will drain her of her spirit. At Brown, a course on "Death and Dying" forced us to confront our own demons about losing life; for as in the rest of pure medical practice, it is not "Physician, heal thyself," but "Physician, know thyself." In the combined liberal arts/premedical program from which I graduated from at Brown Medical School (and that still endures as *The Program in Liberal Medical Education*), I read about the body and soul from the great body of literature written by other human beings reaching to come to terms with the universal pain of knowing we will die—but not always how or when, or how we will deal with what knowledge we are given ahead of time. I followed gifted hematology/oncologists, those physicians who see leukemias and other cancers, and treat but cannot cure all, and watched them care for those from childhood to older age. They worked wholly, their hearts open and with hurt at times, but they did not flinch from patients. They chose medicine knowing loss and joy would always need to be faced in this profession, just as being human requires. These doctors remembered they did not control life or death, and that freed them to do their best and live with it. I left with a sense that being given the opportunity and highest trust of human beings to be present at the most intimate moments of their lives, whatever the specialty, is a chance to serve beyond words.

Dickens wrote about those who "are there from the lying-in to the laying out"; I chose this in family medicine. I felt I had been shown how to step up with guts to all these plates. Surgeons open and close the body in the stark, antiseptic atmosphere of the operating theater; they train a spotlight onto one isolated human section and see it, touch it, for what are only moments when measured over the course of a life. Those of us in primary care are allowed to be present from the excitement of the opening to the breathtaking closing of a person's mortal time— the truly greatest show on earth.

Seek and pray for the right way for each patient when death braves life. Do not just lift your pen and order some "thing." Lift your heart. A patient and his family often look to the physician to lead, calmly, with knowledge and understanding of the mind and teaching about the body. People need to be able to lean, even when they feel they know the right path. A doctor can enable people to thread their way through their jungle of choices and fears—and avoidance of this, doing more tests instead of talk, is a failure of both courage and brains in a physician.

It is never the substance of just one life that is changed by the death of another. At the moment of death, a moment that none on earth, including those in medicine, can predict with absolute precision, we are all technically alone—but part of the ritual of life is to be able to feel one bore witness to the passing of a kindred human being into another realm.

Read such as Dylan Thomas's poem, *Do Not Go Gentle Into That Good Night*, or absorb James Joyce's stories of *The Dead* to understand another kind of human end. Let yourself be squeezed against a wall of recognition that "attention must be paid" to Willy Loman in Arthur Miller's *Death of A Salesman.* Attend when someone you love leaves you. Do not retreat from but turn to a patient, a family, when this transition to another sphere occurs; the life force you will feel will astonish, and yes, replenish you. It will seem as miraculous—in a turnabout, simple human way as you touch another to the end—as Michaelangelo's vision of the finger to finger of God and man.

The Irish say the dead are never truly gone, but "just out of the corner of your eye." Hospice literature teaches that in death those moving away are like a ship at the horizon—already looking forward, with godspeed, and able to see the other shore that we cannot. Soon to be just out of our sight.

Keep both death and life in your sight at all times. Revere—honor—both. They are both ours forever. They are both beyond wonder.

Rule #8
Hospitals Are Why Stations

I love hospitals. I always have. And it is a craze with passion. Within their walls move all of what it means to be human: to reach out, rush in, cry, scream, laugh, endure, surrender, snatch back. Stand in confusion. Lose a part of you, gain back hope. Connect or let go. Pray and blaspheme. Curse. Invent. Give praise for a miracle. Wail, for there is a time when only a wail will do. Take the name of your Lord and/or your doctor in vain. Put your trust in another and also learn what you can, and must, do for yourself. Find out what you are made of. Wonder how you will go on—or why you should.

Circulation is the hum of the human body, the system always flowing. So must a hospital be: self-contained movement with purpose, permeated with life-centered energy. Always about to move up and down the stairwells, through the corridors and in and out of the rooms of a hospital is a broad-shouldered power, sometimes swaggering, then a sentinel—akin to the legendary Finn MacCool, the Irish Giant. Armed with his code of honor, he strode through his land determined to fight for the lives of those around him, and his footsteps in battle flung great clumps of earth behind him, creating the space for the providence of lakes and the refuge of the Isle of Man. Never static inside, a hospital stands as a sheltering, whirling hurricane with a clear eye. Dual beauty in duty.

You can feel this strength in the thickess of a hospital's am-
bient air: the idiosyncratic smell of one body after surgery, of
another's sweat before, and the rigid silence without heat when
life leaves, the early edge of decomposition coming...the perfume
of tears, the sucked-in breath of a family's relief, or loss, billow-
ing towards the whiff of "the lipstick sign" on a healed woman
ready to go home...blood avalanches with their unmistakable stink
as they cathartically sail and smash along disintegrating bowel
walls, trying to turn the owner's life inside out...sheets that snap
with the odor of disinfectant...the plastic plates. Alcohol in swabs,
rubber on hands and in tubes, machine metal, all of it merging
into the unmistakable incense that coats the communicants who
arrive on schedule—or thunder in like a flood. Doctors scrub
with holy water and multiple believers gather with them to comfort an unyielding need. A teeming continual service—en masse.

And then, a button is pushed, by a member of the family,
and the beginning of *Brahms' Lullaby* plays throughout the hospital—announcing the birth of a child. This now occurs where I
trained, St. Joseph's Hospital Health Center in Syracuse, New
York. Imagine its effect, as the sweet notes carry the universal
scent of a human newborn. It pulls together all souls who hear it.

A hospital manifests its own character, and it tests that of
others. One wounded warrior enters bearing the design of his
his crest and his struggle, and others stand at the brink of choice:
What shall I do? Why has life brought me here? Even those
who know they will walk out of the hospital, that behemoth
that swallows some people whole, join the chorus of voices
that weave in and out of harmony. All cry out to the hospital—
*Teach me, save me, take me in, let me go. Make sense of pain
that can seem senseless.*

So I will name you as cathedrals: St. Vincent, St. Joseph's,
Providence, Mount Sinai, Beth Israel, Bon Secours (Good Help),
or Bellevue (Beautiful Sight). Sint Lukas Ziekenhuis in Hol-
land; Mater Miserecordia (Mother the Heart of Mercy) in
Dublin; and Hospitalier St. Jean de Dieu (St. Joan of God) in
France. Simply, in Paris—Hôtel-Dieu, the private mansion of
God. All holy places, and all over the world. Wherever I find

you, and need you, I may walk in, or enter on my knees, confess sins and vow repentance—and yet I may never change my ways. I will surrender or strain at your rules. But when my breath is taken away, my heart makes no sound, my limb is cut, my labor truly begins, my child, my wife, my father, myself, any and all shotgun the air with the original message of pain, I will come to your portal as a pilgrim. Wanting to believe. Standing, staring at your enduring necessity, at your sliding doors of humanly stained great glass that "automatically open," I will step over the threshold, no longer the agnostic questioning the religion that goes on within—but knowing it is both important, and true.

A child watched as the women crowded her, slathering her arms with unguent. Petroleum jelly. Her skin fell away like soaked tissue paper. In the car on the way to the doctor she asked, "Is my hair on fire?"

That child was now delirious.

"God, it's midnight and it's still ninety degrees in here. What's her temperature now?"

The mother looked at her sister. "One hundred and four."

The child writhed and heaved the washcloth off her forehead. From her seat next to her child on the couch the mother bent down to retrieve it, wrung it, and then wiped her own face as the girl spewed gibberish sounds. Three days ago she'd come to this rental cottage to show her daughter the same beach where her own father had baptized her with the "holy water of the Atlantic"—where she'd floated in the welcome of the sea, sensing womb-like safety. She'd brought her own water baby. Three minutes ago that baby shook as if God was holding her by the arms, angry with his doll; and she knew he couldn't be. Why? Why this now? Why ever.

"Jesus, Mary, and Joseph—she's burning up. I'm calling another doctor. What the hell was Crowe thinking letting her come home like this?"

Twenty minutes later the mother opened the door to the male stranger. He was dressed in a shirt and tie and introduced himself as his eyes strayed over her shoulder to his patient. He squeezed in next to the child on the sofa.

"She's six, Doctor."

"The bandages?"

"Hot water. To sterilize baby bottles. It was boiling on the stove when we stopped to see her great aunt. On my father's side." The mother sucked in a little air. "She went for ice cream with all her cousins, wanted a glass of water when she came back."

"And those goddamn Phelans think they have to scald every last germ out of the glass," the sister said. She bent to kiss her niece's cheek. "She's such a sweet kid, I think she jumped up to get a towel to wipe her hands on instead of on her sunsuit and hit that damn pot…thank God it didn't hit her face."

The doctor pinned the child gently as he checked her lungs, her heart, her swaddled arms and legs and trunk. He turned to the mother.

"Nine people in that little pantry. I was just inches from her…and not a drop on anyone else," she said. She felt her face hovering and wavy in the heat. The doctor stood and took her hand.

"The burns are infected. She needs to go to the hospital. Now. You've got three choices: Massachusetts General, Floating, or Children's."

The mother remembered her next words as surely as her memory would see that night like a freeze-frame until dementia erased it. "She's only a child. The place for what she is."

My father got a call in New York to join us sooner than the weekend as planned; I began my month in Children's Hospital in Boston. Even as a child I was fascinated by the world into which chance thrust me. The state of the art of burn care then seems archaic now: large wards, with my bed at one of the corners, and embryonic and few antibiotics. I remember a nervous young man attempting to slide a needle into the top of my hand—an intern with an IV. Scant visiting hours even for parents who kept vigil every day, a man and a woman lanced by shock—but from the terrace I was eventually allowed on I could wave at my baby sister. A small boy who had bitten an electrical cord roamed the ward with a fire hole of a mouth. A pretty blonde teenager wheeled around in the solarium with only the thigh remaining of her left leg. I spent the first weeks of my stay wrapped from the neck down, pushing against a foot board to prevent contractures.

My parents brought me a Madame Alexander doll, wind-up clowns, and a gyroscope. How amazing its balance and inner twirl on a string—or not, suddenly. Like life. I saw the hospital as a place apart where prayers storming heaven might not be the difference between needing skin grafts or seeing the singed layers remake themselves on their own; but they couldn't hurt.

I don't believe that being anointed as a patient so young played into my decision to become a doctor, any more than finding out that a distant relative, the only other physician in the family, has a building relic named after him at the remaining innards of what was Boston City Hospital. But who can tell all of that which propels us, our inner mysteries, to what we should do, must do? I do know that a part of me couldn't imagine being here doing anything else: How could one not want to devour how human beings are—inside and out—know the genius of the body, the spirit? Like living twice all the time. How can someone not want to walk through life like that? When I see one of my children, all the pathways and chemicals and orbits making this process possible come to mind at the same time as the beyond-diagram emotions I feel at this miraculous sight. Starting my medical education I obtained the microfiche of my records from Children's Hospital, a name that to this day, in any city there is such a place, connotes the special care of those most dependent. The gentlest holding in our hands. I had to read the notes on my stay because of a compelling scientific interest (what percentage of the burns were third-degree, or second-degree like my Cape Cod sunburn blisters…how did it fit with the "rule of nines" I had now learned to use to estimate such things…) glued to the sense of being pulled back into the fold. The "why" was asked and asked again; but the different possible answers could lie quiet in the wonder of the hospital. It is that "magnificent obsession" that I try never to lose in my days as a doctor—and that I stubbornly maintain is necessary for anyone who would work in a hospital as physician. Drawn to the work. Without question. An apostle of serving in one's midst. And my time as a patient, tiny as my scars are, gave me some added response to be used, unspoken, to a patient's "Why?"

Nothing fully, decently human will be wasted as a physician; having all the answers, especially to "why" is not needed. One must only be open to all kinds of questions.

"I'm afraid I didn't quite hear your question."

"How long have you had the lump in your breast?"

"It's not really a lump."

That was not what it said on her admitting papers. "Mrs. Lorraine Gilders. 47. Large mass right breast. To undergo biopsy and treatment." And the "Mrs." being the wife of the head of this floor, S-2, the chief of the Private Teaching Service—Surgeon David H. Gilders, M.D.

I was on the next day after being on call, and too hungry to look forward to a debate. I wanted to transcribe the "history of the present illness" concisely and rapidly, and I needed to accomplish this in as perfect a form as possible to have it pass muster at rounds. With the famous Dr. Gilders.

July, the air conditioning in the hospital was overwhelmed, but the two-bed room still had a faint off odor that seemed more than I was used to in this heat wave. I shifted a tad in my white coat to be sure it wasn't piggy-backed on me. I had changed scrubs about 4 am after Mr. Norinksi, one of our repeat offenders, had puked on me and the ER, barely taking time to announce it with a loud whiskey-fueled belch. As my mother would say, he'd "been meaning to bring that up," and I hadn't perfected my dodge-ball maneuver in time.

"Mrs. Gilders—how would you describe it?"

She smoothed the hospital gown over her chest. "Hardly anything. I mean, I can barely see it. My husband just thinks I should have it checked."

That funny smell was still there. Even with my allergies and clogged nose.

"Any pain with it?" She shook her head, looking down.

"And you've had it how—"

"Oh, just a few weeks. Yes. Just two. About."

I rubbed my eyes, finished the routine inquiries, and told her I would do the physical now. Normocephalic (normal shape and size head), eyes (fundi), ears (otolaryngeal), thyroid gland, stethoscope on the back and listen to deep breaths…breast exam…soaked gauze pad…

"How long have you had this?"

"Not very long."

Right breast. Five by six centimeter hole in the skin, fungating—the diameter of an orange splayed out like a cauliflower. Visible now, the smell was nauseating. It oozed pus at its core, rotting through the skin and almost down to what I presumed was the chest wall muscle layer, carved out. Hard as stone. Just as immovable.

Nothing.

Metastatic cancer of the breast, longstanding, no question about it. But more additional questions than the lush auburn hairs on her head. How could her husband let it go this long? Did they sleep together? Did he give a damn about her? How did she stand the smell, especially alone with it after a shower, getting changed for bed? Did she close her eyes, never look down, afraid she'd fall and cry out? What the hell was the matter with her, *why* did *she* wait so long? Did she want to die?

I searched her face. The beauty of its design resilient.

"I think I forgot to tell you my mother died of breast cancer."

The answer. I watched my mother, they tortured her, it didn't make any difference, I'm doomed so I might as well pretend I'm normal as long as I can—take your pick. And all bulging under the seminal "why"—Why me?

Why any of us.

But why did Mrs. Gilders come in then? She was never able to talk to any of us about what was truly in front of her; she may have done so with her husband. He never addressed the nonsurgical part of her care with his trainees. I wondered about their history together, whether from some blind cave inside she spoke any anger at him by rendering him powerless in her case. It's still my life; you're not going to cut me again. She waited to come in until she'd made her decision clear—and in the hospital she claimed sanctuary.

There are many cases where the "what" is simple and clean—classic gall bladder colic, pneumonia, gout. Identifying the "what," the medical categories, does answer why. Just not all of it every time. Being on the lookout for all of it is seeing the entire iceberg, trying to avoid fatal collisions. The diabetic is admitted in near coma because his blood sugar is peak-climbing to ten times normal; but why is this the second or third "revival" of this performance, indeed, with several repeat co-stars, in this particular body? Does he not understand how to take his medicines; is the family member in charge of seeing that he eats right letting the patient down? Is one of his other prescribed medicines fouling up the works?

And as doctors what part of our work can we improve? We can intercept some of the other factors, point the way to other support. Such is the power entrusted to us with our medical licenses that we can do much with just one phone call, one order. See the whole person in a complex existence and try to polish one facet. Why not?

People come to hospitals searching for saints—and not seeing that value also in themselves. They give money for new wings of these buildings even before donating to their churches. They pray for redemption when hooked up to the flickering votive lights of heart monitors, and worship our ritual ceremonies of blood taking, the graven radiology images, and the blessings with Betadine before being opened up to surgical sacrifice. Our pronouncements carry the weight of their world: "critical," "on the danger list," "now stable." More present to them each day than the security alerts of the nation. They need to know the books, the training, from which we preach if we expect them to keep faith.

Their lives may be *The Lives of the Saints.*

Today I am the one who puts her earrings on. I want her to look like herself. I need her to look like herself when I look at her.

"And what brings you in today?"

Okay. No Marx Brothers smart retort or any dumb joke replies like "A Humvee." Why is this the first response that comes to my mind considering our situation? The young lady is only doing her job; and I need to do my new one.

"RECEPTIONIST" hangs over her head. Fingers—*That's a French manicure. Why does the curse of being a trained observer have to follow me in here now, like in elevators*—poised over her keyboard—*she looks like she took piano lessons from the way she holds her fingers—*she keeps smiling at my mother. Who then turns smiling to me, also looking for her answer.

This is an eighty-four-year-old white female, in her usual state of good health until her brain decamped... "She's been quite agitated at home, barely sleeping, roaming the house all night. Much worse this week." *Try much worse this year.* "In the kitchen, at the stove, fiddling with all the faucets, including the bathtub. I called the hospital, and they said to bring her to the emergency department to be screened for admission to the Geriatric Psychiatric Unit." *Actually I called, finally, because my closest woman friend **and** my doctor said, "Look, it's okay, you've done all you*

*can. Really. You can't keep doing this alone…you have three chil-
dren to take care of… and yourself."* So much simpler to tell
another to do this; I'd done it myself, feeling I was as empathetic
as humanly possible. Of course. I'm the overachiever.

My mother and I sit, holding hands, watching the mounted
television in the waiting room. I straighten an earring. We both
lose track of time and thoughts. *Television—Man-Made
Alzheimer's—Five Hundred Cable Channels Inside. And Now
Available: "On Demand."*

The nurse smiles at my mother as she wraps the blood pressure cuff around her arm, and my mother, of course, smiles back.
The same knockout one that brought my father over to her in that
restaurant in New York City; the same one in damn near every
picture taken of her. Perhaps the last human reflex to
depart the brain.

We form a smile ring. The nurse says "Dr. Warner will be
right in," "right" once again part of Einstein's original theory of
relativity. But it doesn't matter because we are relatively safe.
We are at the hospital.

My mother knows her first name, answers "Here" when
asked if she knows where she is, turning her head to me or the
doctor like a contestant on a quiz show before she answers each
question. A lot of prize money riding on it. She doesn't know
the "correct" response to "Why are you here?" pleading only
"You know."

The "designated mental health professional" (which prompts
the question about our collective amateur status) and her trainee
take my mother to a separate room to interview her "alone." They
eye me and my initial move to go with her as if I had kidnapped
her, kept her hostage, and wanted to control her mind. If only. Dr.
Warner and I are alone in the room.

"I never really believed I would be on this side of the white
coat one day."

Dr. Warner stops writing on his clipboard. A reasonable
smile, but no answer.

"All those years I sat where you are, on that stool. Spoke chapter and verse, from memory. Gave orders. And then—you change places. You're the care "taker" not the care "giver.""

He looks up. Probably about thirty-five years old, earned surety and professionalism, but still quiet.

"Thank you—you've been genuinely kind," I say. "It's just so strange to watch you helping us."

The brain trust return my mother. The "head" one asks if she could speak with me alone. How thoughtful; my turn of the screw.

"She's really quite demented, you know." *You doctor. You idiot.*

"I know."

"You could have brought her in sooner."

"I know that, too. But I was committed to keeping her home with me, with her family, as long as possible. Bringing her in to stamp her official diagnosis on a chart wasn't going to stop the loss of her mind. We tried all the meds supposed to put the brakes on, and they failed. Besides—some of the words she made up were quite beautiful." *Put that in your pipe and smoke it, as my mother would say right now to you if she could remember it.*

That's why we came to the hospital. That day. You make your way to the majesty of the building when you don't know what else to do, where else to turn. You knock on the doors and it should take you in—like a cathedral on a hill, drawing its people to it, a family never refusing. Come in, sit down, pray if you want to, take part in our communion, find solace in our order. Nothing about being human is foreign to us, for we struggle like you. And we find and share stunning hope. Within our walls are your first and last rites, your birthright. Your ransom has been paid.

Hospitals have become, to the Byzantine money-changers of our flailing healthcare system, quick "way stations": short-stay units, length-of-stay comparisons, you can't stay here. Any longer. With the addition of grace, "Sisters" (as the British call nurses, and a term of deep respect woman to woman) have also become "high priestesses"; we could use more even if they work only part-time, because their sentience is with them at all times. Despite the craziness of the system the best of all consecrators remain grounded in their common human frailty. Still, we must find a way to keep hospital pews welcoming and the great doors open—for the religion within is what we need to have.

My math teacher in high school was besotted with his subject, and through his gifts, the vision of his love, we eagerly became likewise obsessed. Mathematics created its own pure universe, and was "as close as man comes to God." Kurt Gödel, a contemporary of Einstein's, showed there were mathematical statements that were true but unprovable. This is what you work with. Timeless truths both within and beyond reach—beauty surpassing explanation. I went on to medical school and came to see that approach as the science, center, and soul of medicine.

In the Episcopal cathedral in Victoria, British Columbia, sits an uncommon, unforeseen joy. You have to look up to see it. Alighted on one of the supports of the nave is a stone nest and carving of a bird: the "Robin Pillar," a sculpture done in tribute to the wee creature for whom all work raising the building ceased until all its eggs were hatched. Medieval cathedrals were designed so high to reach closer to God, as a tiny flesh-and-blood bird can. In flight. In the midst of the hospital, in the time between heartbeats, listen for the grace note, the bird's song, of a finite life—a life that can change in a moment—coursing through the silence and the light between heaven and earth.

That's why we're here.

Rule #9
How To Use Medical Lingo

"Define the course and relations of the radial nerve."

Crap.

"This will constitute 40 percent of your grade on this test."

Double crap. This is the final, which means this may be my last official act as a first-year medical student before I've even had time to expel the smell of formaldehyde on my hands.

Okay. Think. For four months you had those hands in the hallow of another's body because she gave you that gift. This chance. Don't let her down; she trusted you to do it. To bring forth something vital from her death. And you had those hands right on this nerve. Remember how you got here (besides the God-given ability to score well on standardized tests which you parlayed into that undergraduate scholarship…)

"We should name her."

"But her head's still covered, and her eyes. How can we know what to call her?"

The four of us stand like a secret service around the gurney in the anatomy lab. Then Kevin, the crew jock—broad-shouldered as well as brilliant—touches her shoulder.

"They're not going to let us open her brain or touch her eyes until the end, when we know what the hell we're doing on the most precious parts. That's why all we got to do today was make three big incisions on her belly and look inside. But she shouldn't have to wait that long to be rechristened from who she was in her real life." His Broadway grin lights up his face. "Hey—maybe she had a great sense of humor. She willed herself here. Let's call her 'Shop'."

Margaret squints at him. "Looks like we've already found the asshole."

"No. Really. Think…every day before we leave we're supposed to fold any opened skin back into place. She'll know we're being careful because we're closing up 'Shop'." Kevin looks at her hooded face, and all of ours. "Because she is still one of us."

Our textbook of anatomy might have an introduction that put it "When a student is assigned to a cadaver or object, he (*sic*) assumes responsibility for its proper care. He will find the subject already preserved or embalmed, the arteries occasionally injected with a (red) coloring matter…the whole body has been kept moist…it is the duty of the dissector to uncover only the parts on which he is engaged….." But luckily at Brown our professors were picked for their ability to show us form as well as model that all our "parts" were to be "engaged" with this "whole body"—and we had been carefully chosen for our interest in honing that.

"…The radial nerve is the main continuation of the brachial plexus and has its origin from the spinal cord as branches of each nerve root from the C5/T1 level…after leaving the axilla it moves medially to laterally along the spiral groove of the humerus…. bifurcates into a sensory and motor branch…the latter becoming the posterior interosseous, which passes deep to the supinator muscle under the arcade of Frohse…the sensory branch travels superficial to the extensor tendons of the thumb, where it ends supplying most of the dorsal surface of the hand…"

So what's the purpose of all this? What difference does it make if you can describe from memory how this nerve is born, what it scoots by, snakes around and who it travels with; the names it assumes in all the particulars of its journey; and how this story ends? Why dissect a human body—why not see it in computer-assisted "virtual cross-section"? Sadly, there are some schools where the latter is all there is, technology being more bountiful than cadavers—because for those who seek to understand the mystery and genius of that legal and secular temple, there is no full substitute for being inside. It imbues one with the requisite awe, beyond imagined ken; and this sense of its sacred form can, must, then abide with you for the rest of your days. In a place as deep as those you have explored in another.

And the language we use as doctors should be as precise as using a scalpel to gently tease away the covering of the brain.

"Mom—wake up! They need you!"

My son and daughter, one on either side of me, are leaning into my face, yelling quietly in the way that only two early adolescents can when speaking to a parent: the hiss order. They are extremely close to me at this moment as we are sardined into the middle section of the six-across seating of a Boeing 747. Speeding 600 miles an hour over the Arctic Circle.

"They need a doctor!"

I look up, having been dozing with my shoes off and a blanket over my knees. The in-flight (we are fleeing home) movie just ended, I misted up at the end with the parent and child reunion, and I am now aiming for sleep so I don't count EVERY MINUTE of claustrophobic prison (how does my six-foot-two son stand it) that remains until landing. The chief steward—the Brits are in charge of our aeroplane—is scanning the huddled mass in second class.

I get up, hold my breath in to get out of my lane, and escape, simultaneously dragging the corner of the blanket as it stuffs itself into one of my clogs when I try to jam them back onto swollen feet. Large plaid toilet paper. The steward examines my trail as I introduce myself.

"Oh good—I'm so glad it's a girly doctor!" he says, leaning close. "The lady has a female problem, you know."

Yes she does; she and her husband. Increasing vaginal bleeding, eight days post-partum; returning home after visiting her parents in England. Sketchy prenatal care and a midwife home birth on *this* side of the Atlantic, with "pretty much no complications—but then this is our first child." The new family—Ms. Claire Hardy, Mr. David Luckenbill, and baby Agnes—are now ensconced in first class so the mother can lie flat with her dizziness.

"Here's our emergency kit." The steward gives me the smile that got him the job, tinged with terror.

It's slim pickings—but I packed my brain in carry-on, and there's a stethoscope and blood pressure cuff in the little aid suitcase. The patient's has only intermittent cramping, no chills so I know she can't have any significant fever as the flip side, and she can tell me how big the clots are, when they got worse, and how many pads she's going through per hour. Her heart rate isn't overly accelerated even with her worry. Her blood pressure is not low; her abdomen's soft. She's okay at the moment.

She and her husband go to the bathroom, I hold the baby, and then mother returns with a progress report. This time fewer cramps and almost no clots; so far, so good. Not as dizzy and less bleeding now that she's been lying down. She relaxes and our steward squats down beside me.

"The captain would like you to speak to the ground medical team. He has them on the radio."

I sit down in the purser's chair behind the pilot and co-pilot. They are charming, pros, and instruct me on how to use the two-way headset—and it's international showtime.

"This is Dr. Winifred in Greenland. Tell me about the patient."

"This is a twenty-seven-year-old female, gravida one, para one, traveling after an apparently uncomplicated NSVD...

past medical history negative...no signs or symptoms to suggest endometritis...pulse eighty-four and regular...not sallow or icteric...abdomen without masses or tenderness, no hepatoslenomegaly, normoactive bowel sounds ...no pelvic exam possible, obviously, but last large clot was now thirty-five minutes ago."

"Do we need to bring the plane down for an emergency landing?"

"No. I believe I can keep her stable off her feet."

"Great. Thanks." The pilot echoes that—"Even if I didn't understand all that stuff you spit out."

Thank you, teachers at Brown, and Charlie and everyone like him, and Mum and Dad for giving me the conscience and heart to take my work seriously and my vision of God for blessing me with the brains to do this job—and thank you, medical lingo. We're thirty thousand feet in the air over the North Pole and Dr. Winifred can't eyeball Ms.Hardy or Mr.Luckenbill or baby Agnes; and Dr.Winifred and I literally can't see each other— *but*—Dr. Winifred has the whole picture. The language I speak to her is designed to send instant detailed information by brain wire. It's verbal anatomy and physiology, prognosis and plan. Scientific shorthand. It is how a doctor learns to think in an organized fashion with structure. That's what medical lingo is designed for: Learn to collect and collate specific findings from history, examination, and tests, subjective and objective information, and transmit that to yourself or to a colleague. Across town or a continent, or to a fellow physician picking up one of your charts to treat your patient on your day off, medical language is documentation for intelligent work. Yes, it can be bastardized as a legal tool—but this parlance is primarily for precise communication for care. To only be used when appropriate.

I walk back to check on my patients. Mother is nursing her baby, and all systems are in harmony. When our madonna and child later sleep, I spend the rest of the flight calming Father with non-medical lingo explanations and reassurance about what is going to happen next—never mind for the next twenty-one years, at least. Complete, real family medicine. Airborne.

My father would stand at the door of my room when I was teenager, watching me clean it up, and say: "A cluttered room is a cluttered mind." (German heritage, born in Brooklyn in 1899—covert natural master of Feng Shui.) So I say a cluttered mind is a clumsy—or worse, crummy—doctor.

To be a "compleat," an excellent doctor you must have easy facility with at least two languages: your birth one and that of medicine (additional linguistic talent is an immeasurable bonus with our patients from all over our planet). You must be fluent in each of the first two, easily slip back and forth between them even in mid-sentence if required, and think and write in both. And you must catch yourself immediately whenever you keep speaking the one the patient doesn't understand. Staying in "medical speak" mode is either (1) ignorant—being so to the patient because you don't know any better and/or because of deficient intelligence, or (2) deliberate—because you need a barricade due to your own fears and/or because you really don't like patients, or (3) one of the possible combination/permutations of (1) and (2). All of these mandate seeking help for your medical career. Or leaving—if it's too late to direct you to more suitable schooling.

In the television show, *The West Wing*, the president's wife is (we finally have come a long way, even if it's only in the mind of a scriptwriter) a physician. She retreats into detailed, unable-to-break-as-a-layperson code when one of the advisors is going over how he wants her to handle announcing that the President has multiple sclerosis. She's in crisis. Her use of medical lingo as a weapon of self and family protection is understandable, but it's still obnoxious. The advisor sends this first lady the same look that a patient has a right to give you if you play the "doctor talk" card with them: "Look. We're in this together. Do you want to help me here, work with me, or what? I can always walk out"—and that's just what the advisor does, reluctantly, because of dead-end frustration.

Resistance to using medical language beautifully and with proper timing also seems so sad because of the inherent music in the words, the way they illuminate what they are designed to describe, as notes on a page do for a pianist. Practicing technique is just as critical for a physician—as is delight in perfecting her ability to perform. Because both musicians and surgeons spends years learning to inculcate physical memory in their hands, so must those who use their hands to do physical diagnosis: learning how to detect a torn nerve is as critical as knowing how to sew the ragged ends back together. (A classic injury to our friend the radial nerve, presenting with hand weakness, is from a mid-shaft fracture to the humerus that cuts through that electrical cable as it goes by. Index of suspicion goes up when a drunk can tell you he remembers leaning his arm over a chair and then falling over—but he can't tell you how many chairs were involved). All doctors and musicians must be trained "athletes," and all must know how to communicate with their audience.

"Dolce," "allergro" on the page of a symphony score; "acctabulum," "speculum" in a medical dictionary. They exist to bring others into the beauty of what we do and should love. Latin, Greek. Acetabulum meaning "vinegar cup," denoting the shape of the hip socket. Speculum for "looking glass," an instrument that enables you to see inside a hidden alcove, whether the ear canal or that for birth. Imagine the less coldly clinical effect on a woman if you explain why you're sticking that shoe-horn shaped thing between her legs, especially if you've just been introduced. Looking up these words can help a student remember them, and then teach them to patients when indicated. The example used need not be as dramatic as our anatomy professor, the distinguished poster boy for what an intimidating, charming male genius looks like, who impressed on us what "spina bifida occulta" stands for by mentioning that he diagnosed his third wife with it when they were dancing— "it" being a gap where a vertebral body or two fail to form a complete ring around the spinal cord. It can be undetectable by symptoms or appearance, so you have to press low and firmly to feel it. But you can explain what those annoying stool cards times three are for: checking for occult blood. "Occult"—hidden to the naked eye. Every opportunity for learning counts.

People want to know what's going on. They want to understand what the body—theirs—does. Some want more information than others; you can read this on their faces, or just ask them and verify. How do you feel in a foreign country where you don't speak the language? I know Americans in France who just run for the nearest MacDonald's; if you keep patients in dark silence about what "lipid" means, why shouldn't they reach for the same thing and foul up their diet too? And tell them what "fasting" means, and why they have to and how long they have to go without intake except water to get a valid measurement. When some reply, "But I'll faint," remember humor: "Hey, as soon as they pull that needle out of your arm you can eat that breakfast you brought. Just don't bring doughnuts." Just don't leave a patient feeling as Lord Byron wrote about a fellow poet: "I wish he would explain his Explanation."

Letters lined up as words were not built to form a barricade, whatever the country of origin. As physicians we aren't given the power of speech to keep people out and to distance ourselves from knowing we will probably, inevitably, one day be on the other side of sickness. Baseball legend Satchel Paige once said, "Don't look back. Something might be gaining on you." Well, just relax—imponderable mortality gains a tiny bit every day we exist. So live in the present and explain to patients and anyone else close to you why you're blabbing about something the way you are. As Claude Bragdon, a turn of the 20th century architect and ponderer wrote: "Health and disease, thought and emotion, are communicable, contagious." Truly.

Attainable.

Patients are also intelligent people, often too courteous to interrupt us when we treat them as otherwise. It's not an altogether bad trend that over the years they have felt more comfortable instructing those who need it in proper etiquette. The great teachers were way ahead of us once again: "This is all very fine, but it won't do—Anatomy—Botany—Nonsense! Sir, I know an old woman in Covent Garden who understands botany better, and as for anatomy, my butcher can dissect a joint full and well."— Thomas Sydenham (1624-1689), M.D.

When you are in medical school and you're keeping your head down to survive one oncoming test after another, sometimes you think this can only get worse. But *it does get better.* From the beginning to the end of your lifelong learning as a physician you should be enthralled with what comes at you. And that will make it easy to hold onto it to absorb it—and then teach it, pass it on, especially to those you are serving.

And if you're organized, because you want to have "an uncluttered mind" and you are classically trained, your approach to the patient will also help you remember what you need to. This is the only way that excellent primary care is done. They say God, and/or the Devil, is in the details, and so sometimes are the headaches when you are trying to slalom your way to the answer(s)—but we have analgesia for all that. Think straight. Line up the human body's reflex responses; remember. Bang the bejesus out of something, and it will thicken to protect itself, whether it's the bottom of your foot (a callus), or the wall of your heart from uncontrolled blood pressure (left ventricular hypertrophy) stretch something and it will hurt when it takes up too much space in the neighborhood: gas trapped in your intestine, or a pimple in the skin. The nature of blood when it slows down is to clot: good when we draw blood from your vein or you get a cut and put pressure on it—bad when it hits a traffic jam in your narrowed arteries and forms a clump and all hell breaks loose downstream in the organ waiting for the oxygen those red cells carry. See the similarities in the old and the young and their clever if unintended disguises. The newborn and the grandparent can both present with pneumonia that wears only confusion and "they just don't look right" because their body can't assemble fever, cough and sputum. And you better believe the mother or any other family member who accompanies this patient and tells you this. *They know.* Patients don't always have to take notes on the above, but a medical student and doctor better do so.

Stalk the path of microscopic events. Be able to see at that level of detail how cells are pioneers crossing the divide of a wound to close the edges of the continents. Visualize the invasion of the army of sepsis on all its fronts. Learn that inflammation may be the initial common pathway for all sorts of conditions and diseases, adding more all the time: asthma, coronary artery syndromes, rheumatoid arthritis. As you understand in medical lingo, help your patients understand in their language.

But all the medical lingo in the world won't help you or those who come to your office if you have a sloppy mind. You can call that cough "bronchitis," but it will be a wastebasket diagnosis if you're throwing the different causes of it (allergies or new asthma/smoke exposure/early heart failure/sneaky infection) into a big brain can because you didn't take the time to get a real history over a timeline. If the patient's pain is changing, going in the wrong direction, think like those pathogens you memorized, and their schedules—they're busy every minute. Don't wait to diagnose a wound infection until you see the white of pus in that site. Otherwise your treatment can fail, (because each of the above needs a different strategy) and maybe the patient won't die (aren't both of you lucky), but they'll be sicker, longer, than they had to be. Take full pride in your work. Whatever the kind of infection, make sure you know the right drug for the right bug—you should use the knowledge that the germs that congregate in the skin don't usually reside in the lungs—and different ones sit in the mouth, especially if the wound is from a human bite (yes, this can happen out of the boxing ring). Don't just throw a big sponge at everything.

Know the natural history of a disease, condition, and all its biorhythms. In your imagination, go home with your patient at night. Hear that bark that comes in nervewracking fits, dry and useless hacking that's forceful enough to bang eyeballs out of sockets. That's the asthma cough, the one that still often kills because it steals breath in the dark—and doctors don't see it.

Where I schooled and trained we were not allowed to present a patient with an "injured ankle." We were expected to have asked that patient such details as the mechanism of injury ("Did you step in a hole and hear a crack?), done a thorough physical exam to check for "point tenderness" (which can be a preliminary "mental xray" because palpating directly over compromised bone can feel to the injured like the doctor has pushed a button of pain), and checked the orthopedic system higher up in the skeleton knowing that force can be transmitted upwards (even if the patient is too focused on the worst hurt to be able to tell you whether his hip also doesn't feel right). You were expected to stretch to the utmost to give the deepest level of diagnostic accuracy for every point along the way. It was the same with a "sore knee." From what? In which part, or how many of the parts of the knee simultaneously? The knee is the single most complicated joint in the body—it is thrilling to know its components and their interaction and weaknesses, and your enthusiasm for both science and serving means that you figure that out.

Make your mind reach the subtleties. Thyroid disease is not only more common in women, but a subset of it comes from inflammation where the body misidentifies its own tissue as foreign and makes antibodies to it. There are simple additional blood tests to find this if you "care to," and it affects what dose of medicine is then the best. Accessing this data bank does become easier to do with practice, and hopefully the algorithms an experienced doctor uses like quicksilver to come to diagnostic choices will only be aided—but never replaced—by computers because the ineffable art that can turn the decision on a dime is innately human. The communication "interface" is different—on both sides. Don't act like a machine. Whether doctors treat people from within on an operating table or from without in an exam room, they must each have the same deep respect for the process that is due the patient.

"Mr. Goldberg's on the phone for his lab results."

"Let me see the chart." He's a new patient and I want to compare the ones in his old records with the blood we drew yesterday.

"Mr. Goldberg. Your fasting blood sugar is above the current recommendations for normal."

"It's never been high before."

I look at the pages again to make sure I read them correctly. "Unfortunately, it has been going back over the last two years. It puts you in the range for diabetes and you know that runs in your family. And with your history of heart disease and the way your cholesterol profile is leaning, you've got more of those cardiac risk factors we talked about."

"Why didn't the other doctor tell me all this?"

Uncomfortable moment. There again but for God's grace go I in the shoes of another human being, this time the previous physician. But the process to keep your eye on, what we all have a right to expect, is not whipping through the results of tests. Mr. Goldberg's last chemistry profile has a scribble on it that reads "Not too bad." Arrgh. The blood test to measure how often his blood sugar has been normal in the last three months (which means the doctor had in his mind the possibility of diabetes) is definitely abnormal, and the handwritten note next to it (for the nurse to tell the patient) says "worsened somewhat." What exactly does that mean? I can't find a previous level to compare. And the lipid tests have been out of range, not miserably, but still definitely, for three years, and the sign-off is "Good." This just stinks. Don't do the test unless it could change the diagnosis or treatment (and thus the patient's *future*), and then use it when it does. Read the entire radiology report; there is information from a colleague on the patient's team who dictated it because it might make a difference in how you put together a plan for the patient. Bluntly put: All these little outrageous slings and arrows constitute hidden but true "mini-malpractice," and this we can fix so there's no "crisis" for either side of the medicine table. Over the course of a lifetime, small numbers that are off do add up—badly. The level of blood sugar that defines diabetes keeps being lowered because earlier diagnosis and treatment prevents complications and affects both the number and the type of days in lives. Tell patients why you want to keep a close rein, with them, on the best blood pressure readings; and what the newest thinking (which is continually tweaked) is about the ideal way to prevent cardiovascular disaster. "Attention must be paid" at all times.

When a physician is in the presence of another human being, she is in the presence of "genius": what the patient knows about himself and how the body is designed. Research leads us to more and greater medical information, but we must always keep in mind how much we don't know. Only God and the baby really know what moment it is "due"; science is still searching for the exact sequence that triggers labor. Leave behind the idea of perfection when attacking the dust bunnies in your living room so you have energy to use your attention to detail where it counts. This is the bigtime. If you're gifted and want to be a doctor with all your molecules, and your obsessive compulsiveness is driving you and everyone around you bonkers, remember we have medicines for that. And then remember all of the above.

Joseph Campbell, the stellar mythologist and teacher, writes about "The Hero's Journey." We are all on that quest—the urge to live the best, right, life for each soul. There is direction in many ways. In medicine there are clear signposts along the path both for those who strive to enter this field and those who enter to find the physician. These clues are written in medical lingo in this part of the world, and the mode of thought, the state of the mind they engender can make all the difference in the journey of a life.

That's why doctors talk the way we do.

Rule #10
Don't Break Your Own Rules

"She's probably just in a coma."

"How do you know?"

"That's what her regular doctor sent her in with."

"Why would she be in a coma?"

"Maybe she had a stroke, or forgot how many sleeping pills she took and overdosed by accident, or cracked her head in the bathtub and has had a slow leak of blood pancaking under her skull. Meals on Wheels called the police when they couldn't get in, then the cops called the doctor and she came in by ambulance. And don't ask me how long she's been like this. We were unable to get any further history from the patient." The last stanza in singsong.

Stephen Laffond and I are standing outside one of the "critical patient" rooms in our emergency department. He's the second-year resident on call and I'm the novice. Allan DeSimone is the senior ER resident, and he's just filled in Stephen on our next admission of the day: Mrs. Olivia Augustine, seventy-eight years old, brought in unresponsive. Paramedics found her on the floor of her apartment.

Stephen looks at DeSimone. "Couldn't get any history, huh? Did you call the family?"

"Apparently they aren't breaking her door down too often, and they don't answer their phone. Look—Walden's her doc and he gave me a list of her meds and allergies. He thinks she's probably just had a stroke because of her age. She's stable. And she's all yours now."

DeSimone wheeled away and I looked at Stephen. "Is he always like this?"

"Well, he's at the end of his shift, but he's usually snide." He handed me the clipboard. "Right now the patient's better off with us."

We took Mrs. Augustine on her stretcher, heart monitor at her feet, up in the elevator and tucked her into a hospital bed. I held the orders sheet and history and physical forms in my hand and sat down.

"Okay. Phyllis—put down what we know and I'll see if she has any old records here. I doubt she's got a significant subdural hematoma snaking over her brain because there isn't any sign of trauma, but maybe she's a closet little-old-lady drinker because she's lonely, and fell when she passed out. We'll get some xrays anyway. She's breathing on her own—so far, so good. She's only on a thyroid med and iron, but she's not pale and doesn't look like she's edematous, so I'm not sure anemia or not enough thyroid hormone replacement explains all this. And she's not on any blood pressure pills, so we better be careful about it just being a stroke. Do the whole physical and the routine admit orders with a drug screen and page me when you're done."

I did. I couldn't find any focal neurological signs pointing to a specific area of brain malfunction. The "routine" orders in those days included a chest film, and the same full blood work and urine screens on everyone—and this was two years before we had CT scanners. The complete chemistry profile tested for all the usual kidney and liver, blood sugar, thyroid, pancreas, blood mineral and electrolyte (including salt) tests. I added cultures to rule out infection and did a spinal tap to check for encephalitis or incipient meningitis even though she didn't have any skin stigmata for one of the most common types, and her vital signs were all normal with no fever.

The blood work came back that afternoon. Mrs. Augustine's calcium level was in the toilet—and that chemical imbalance was why she was non compos mentis. Medical records finally unearthed her past history and when a surgeon had removed her thyroid gland—so long ago that you couldn't trace the scar in her neck skin folds—apparently her parathyroid glands had accidentally come along for the ride (not a sign of poor technique, since the glands can be almost impossible to identify and vary in number from person to person). The surgeon had checked her labs post-operatively just as he should have, and she was put on calcium replacement.

But she wasn't taking it, either because she ran out, forgot, or it wasn't followed by Dr. Walden. And apparently this part of her history slipped his mind when he gave his diagnosis over the phone, either because he wasn't organized or he slipped into a conclusion. But we followed our system of approach and our training to think it through for ourselves and checked every possibility.

We gave her calcium—and she woke up. And she talked our ears off, in the best way.

She didn't slip through our hands.

The rules of admission, of the most current evidence-based medicine, have changed since then, but *the rule* hasn't: Don't break your own rules. Don't cheat on asking the same inclusive history questions referable to the presenting symptoms and "complaint" of the patient—especially if she can't tell you the whole story. Don't scrimp on the physical. Put it all together: The diagnosis, *the vital connection,* can turn on one moment, one look, one phrase. One feeling; one thought. One choice. Do the job the same way even if nobody is ever going to check your work, as if you were working in a closet and there was no such thing as peer review and "quality assurance"—which now they do when you call the telephone company. Wondering if your exam is being taped or monitored shouldn't be your benchmark.

Keep up with the advances in medical care, in the ideal ways to manage chronic diseases, like diabetes and heart problems, both rampant in this country and the world. Smart care is exciting care.

But remember information is everywhere: in texts, in charts—in the room. Cutting corners on asking questions or doing the full exam and "getting away with it," either because no harm comes to the patient or no one reads your chart, means you're a dummy. None of us want to see a dummy except on the knee of a ventriloquist.

And this work as a physician should be joyful. Delight in being privileged to "see" the parallel inner universe that the body runs on: the artistry of its twenty-four hour clock, something *always* happening to nourish, repair, relax in provident life. Its rules are a psalter. Revel with it. Hear the music in a patient's accent—and tell them. You can hold that thought with a "medical" one in your mind at the same time. And when you do, something different will happen in that room—something more therapeutic.

You can be an ace and still be funny. That attitude will be as easy to spread as any virus. When you work with patients be human and when you dictate a patient's story, write with verve. You may find your best phrase to describe how high someone's blood pressure climbed is "at its zenith...," and you can take heart together that it's fallen back to earth, normal. And when the patient comes back and his infection is improved on the pill you agreed upon, celebrate in the office: "Isn't it beautiful when modern American medicines work as advertised?" Use your wit and personality and smarts to be a real person with patients—that's what each of us wants when we entrust our lives to another. (You can also write originally in your personal life, like the unattached ophthalmologist I knew who put "SGL DOC" on the license plate of his Porsche convertible.) Don't try to know it all; you never can, and no one likes a God-pretender anyway. As a cardiology professor from Harvard once said to me when I saw, and was shocked, that he was looking up the American Heart Association guidelines for the prevention of subacute bacterial endocarditis (heart valve infection): "That's why they have reference books." He was right. The rules you need to commit to memory and *live* are the ones I've put in this book. This is where the measure of medicine is—not rote recitation.

If something doesn't feel right, it isn't, as true in the work of a physician as in giving your children a sense of ethics, or in choosing whom to marry. Let the loose end, the fact that doesn't fit, niggle at you, make you fidget in your mind, until you put it to rest. Whether it's physiological or personal. If you know a patient is angry, whether at you or how the office system has treated him, go into the room and take care of it before the fiery dragon between you makes it impossible for you both to breathe normally, or think straight. Be direct and kind as you acknowledge the issue—the pricking of the pissed-off balloon is going to be a huge relief on both sides, and then you can take care of the work, the patient, at hand.

When you see patients as too "needy," remember we all are. Flesh and blood are fragile creations. Find balance in your life. Make sure you take vacations—seek out or create your own art, liberally. Love your family. Treat them as well as your patients (no street angel, home devil). Congratulate a patient when she does finally quit smoking, and take comfort in each human victory. It all counts. To do the right thing as a doctor can sometimes mean (as my mother one more time would say) being "tougher than boiled owl"; but there will always be those transcendent moments when a patient will knock you off your feet with what she brings to your life.

Don't change as a human being because of what happens to you in medicine; either as a physician or as a patient. Whatever side of the curtain we are on, we must be steadfast in what we believe is the right thing to do. You can love it with your whole heart and your whole mind and your whole soul, like an old catechism promise, but this doesn't mean dying on the altar of medicine. Speak up—there is to be no human sacrifice on either side of the medical equation.

Plant your mouth for what you believe, for the world must not mistake your courtesy for weakness. All physicians in all specialties can campaign for what we need in medicine now to stop the ruin. We need *time*. Primary care is under siege. A gun at our head shoves us into a new room every fifteen minutes; even better if even faster. I tell patients exactly why this occurs: because the pay per minute for primary medical care is so low. Let this word get out, and out, and out. All patients *need* the kind of medical home that a fine family physician provides—yet the value of being able to do the right care the first time is a "claim denied" by our third party payers. Fewer students chose primary care because of huge medical school debts, the insane work pace, and the sense that their daily patient volume will be counted but they won't be. Let our President or members of the United States Congress follow me in and out of rooms all day. See a real visit with a real patient in real time. Many patient charts are the size of the Manhattan phonebook. It doth not profit any health insurance conglomerate, or Medicare or Medicaid to force a doctor to see people like a money machine—he can only use his eyes and mouth, and brain and heart, so fast. There's that pesky rate-limiting factor. Our (patients, physicians, payers) mutual goals should be profoundly human: Move people to make the changes at home that we tell them about in the office, to take care of the one body that is all they get, to keep themselves out of hospitals except when it is the life-saving place. Game-show-like rapid encounters are "pernicious"—the word means "leading to fatality." They do not "control" healthcare costs, because they don't help us show people how to give themselves health and make it self-renewing. We know how to fix this.

One alternative solution is the trend of doctors opening practices where they do not take health insurance. They have only reasonable overhead, they charge flat fees for the time or type of service—and as they see ten patients a day they do not have to break their own rules of truly being complete physicians helping, connecting with patients. Monetarily this will not work for all. But even with the system we now have, insurance companies can make a difference. Excellent primary care physicians, as with leaders in any discipline, can welcome being paid for performance; those who follow the rules in this book should be. Give me a diabetic with high blood pressure and lousy lipids and I'll put them on the right medicines at the right doses and monitor their chronic diseases according to the state of our art and science; and I'll get them to work with me and come back. But don't you *dare* say I can do that in fifteen minutes. Even the best patient won't be able to reel off all we cover via that rapid transit. Experienced clinicians who bring a lot more brain power into the room (and there is no question a doctor knows a great deal more after residency) should cost more to see—because seeing someone who gets it right the first time, and connects, is transparently more cost and health effective. The third party payers, crowding the party, must accept this; they're spending more and more money on the decorations and the invitations, but they've got goons stationed at the door.

All physicians need to insure that the few but persistent doctors who do not follow the standard of care are brought to account. This is just as much a part of our duty to "First Do No— Do Not Allow This—Harm." How in God's name can a lay person "shop" for the "best" medical care? We as physicians know what the rules are—we must use them with ourselves and then be allowed to use them with our patients. Give us this daily time. The human and dollar costs of this current lunacy are exponential. Don't push our patients out the door—this is pushing ever more good physicians out of the profession.

I am an acknowledged and shameless primary care chauvinist. This is the reason why: *A young woman goes to see a doctor because of nausea. The neurologist wonders if she hit her head and orders a CT scan. The gastroenterologist suggests that she let him put a scope down and take a look at her gut. And the family physician takes a look at her face and asks: "What did you eat last night? Is anyone else in your family sick? Are you worried about exams? And when was your last period?"* I chose to be a family physician because we take all comers and gleefully throw a lasso around it all—and each doctor must find the specialty that is his or her heart's desire.

I am also a chauvinist for the type of education I received at Brown Medical School—its idea, its reality, its future. The right kind of students, those with fire in the core of their souls and seeking to serve, must be found and shown the breadth of humanity, including the humanities; they must be honed as clinicians and as human beings who go out into the world to make a difference; and they must be supported in this work by the healthcare system. I have tried to live this, fallible as we all are, and I don't always come within sight of the Grail. But I do keep where the mark is in my head and heart. I have tried to make it clear in this book of rules. If I have succeeded, it will be clear that all the rules fit together and should not be loosed apart. They are designed to form a ring of beauty and the height of skill—as Frederick Law Olmstead and Calvert Vaux aimed for in their blueprint for Central Park. I hope to point the way along these paths in medicine as Cristo and his wife Jeanne-Claude did with such impact recently with their life art installation "The Gates" in that same landmark and oasis in New York City. This book aims to be unforgettable in its way.

Joseph Campbell also noted that we should all "follow our bliss"—and Brown helped me find mine. This work means everything to me. My way of continuing to understand and follow my bliss is to write such as this:

Attending

I have attended death
Praying first to have the Spirit flow
Through me with the truest words to
Comfort those left behind
And
I have dissected death, both from without
Suddenly without those I loved and
From within, seeing the anatomy of the body

Probing my own invisible mind
And
Grasping for the place where the soul and
The breath of life lie
Knowing no doctor knows Lazarus
For a father can slip from me
And
A heart can stop pulsing
To slip away becoming pure spirit free of thin dust
Free at last to return to its source, to God, as a tide
Belongs to the sea
And
Just as uncontrollably and beyond measure
I have seen a mother let go of a baby
Being born who reaches out with its hands
As it cries alive, Alive
And
So I have attended Life
New and old and struggling and joyous
To be here and blessed to believe
That whosoever believes

Will never die.

Whoever and whatever we deeply love never dies. There is a ninety-two-foot high brick bell tower, Carrie Tower, on the front green of the Brown University campus in Providence, Rhode Island. It was erected in 1904 by a man in honor of his perished wife, his sweetheart. Inscribed at its base are these words, from 1st Corinthians: "Love is strong as death."

To be a doctor—it's the damnedest job in the world. But as the last of my mater's famous words, remember that "As God makes them He matches them." Don't get engaged—don't take the oath of medicine—unless it's your Own True Love. Your commitment needs to be that strong, and large, and as clear as a bell.

A bell that rings for Life.

Sacred Trust
The Ten Rules of Life Death and Medicine

Please send me_____ copy(ies) of *Sacred Trust* at $13.95 each ($18.95 Canadian) plus $5.00 shipping and handling. For each additional, add $2.00 shipping and handling. Washington residents please add $1.24 sales tax per book.

Phone Orders:
425-483-3040
Have your VISA/MasterCard ready.

Fax Orders:
425-483-3098
Fill out this order form and fax.

Email Orders:
sherynhara@earthlink.net

Mail Orders:
Book Publishers Network
P.O. Box 2256
Bothell, WA 98041

Payment—please circle one: Check VISA MasterCard

Name_____Phone_____

Address_____

City/State/Zip_____

Credit Card # _____

Exp. Date_____

Signature_____

www.hollenbeckmd.com